Achieving QTS
Reflective Reader: Primary Professional Studies

Achieving QTS: Reflective Readers

Reflective Reader: Primary Professional Studies
Sue Kendall-Seatter
ISBN-13: 978 1 84445 033 6 ISBN-10: 1 84445 033 3

Reflective Reader: Secondary Professional Studies
Simon Hoult
ISBN-13: 978 1 84445 034 3 ISBN-10: 1 84445 034 1

Reflective Reader: Primary English
Andrew Lambirth
ISBN-13: 978 1 84445 035 0 ISBN-10: 1 84445 035 X

Reflective Reader: Primary Mathematics
Louise O'Sullivan, Andrew Harris, Margaret Sangster, Jon Wild, Gina Donaldson and Gill Bottle
ISBN-13: 978 1 84445 036 7 ISBN-10: 1 84445 036 8

Reflective Reader: Primary Science
Judith Roden
ISBN-13: 978 1 84445 037 4 ISBN-10: 1 84445 037 6

Reflective Reader: Primary Special Educational Needs
Sue Soan
ISBN-13: 978 1 84445 038 1 ISBN-10: 1 84445 038 4

Achieving QTS

Reflective Reader
Primary Professional Studies

Sue Kendall-Seatter

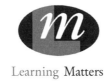

Learning Matters

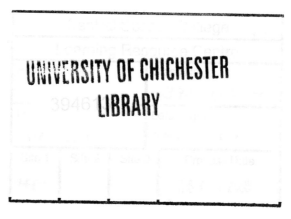

First published in 2005 by Learning Matters Ltd.

British Library Cataloguing in Publication Data
A CIP record for this book is available from the British Library.

ISBN-13: 978 1 84445 0 33 6
ISBN-10: 1 84445 0 33 3

Cover design by Topics – The Creative Partnership
Project management by Deer Park Productions, Tavistock, Devon
Typeset by PDQ Typesetting Ltd, Newcastle-under-Lyme
Printed and bound in Great Britain by Bell & Bain Ltd, Glasgow

Learning Matters Ltd
33 Southernhay East
Exeter EX1 1NX
Tel: 01392 215560
Email: info@learningmatters.co.uk
www.learningmatters.co.uk

Contents

Introduction

The *Reflective Reader* series supports the *Achieving QTS* series by providing relevant and topical theory that underpins the reflective learning and practice of primary and secondary ITT trainees.

Each book includes extracts from classic and current publications and documents. These extracts are supported by analysis, pre- and post-reading activities, links to the QTS Standards, a practical implications section, links to other titles in the *Achieving QTS* series and suggestions for further reading.

Integrating theory and practice, the *Reflective Reader* series is specifically designed to encourage trainees and practising teachers to develop the skill and habit of reflecting on their own practice, engaging with relevant theory and identifying opportunities to apply theory to improve their teaching skills.

The process of educating individuals is broader than the specific areas of educational theory, research and practice. All humans are educated, socially, politically and culturally. In all but a few cases humans co-exist with other humans and are educated to do so. The position of an individual in society is determined by the nature and quality of the educational process. As a person grows up, emerging from childhood into adulthood, their social and political status is dependent on the educational process. For every task, from eating and sleeping to reading and writing, whether instinctive or learnt, the knowledge and experience gained through the process of education is critical. Humans are educated, consciously and subconsciously, from birth. Education is concerned with the development of individual autonomy, the understanding of which has been generated by educational, sociological, psychological and philosophical theories.

The position of the teacher in this context is ambivalent. In practice each teacher will have some knowledge of theory but may not have had the opportunity to engage with theories that can inform and improve their practice.

In this series, the emphasis is on theory. The authors guide the student to analyse practice within a theoretical framework provided by a range of texts. Through examining why we do what we do and how we do it the reader will be able to relate theory to practice. The series covers primary and secondary professional issues, subject areas and topics. There are also explicit links to Qualifying to Teach Standards (QTS) that will enable both trainees and teachers to improve and develop their subject knowledge.

Each book provides focused coverage of subjects and topics and each extract is accompanied by support material to help trainees and teachers to engage with the extract, draw out the implications for classroom practice and to develop as a reflective practitioner.

While the series is aimed principally at students, it will also be relevant to practitioners in the classroom and staffroom. Each book includes guidance, advice and examples on:

- the knowledge, understanding, theory and practice needed to achieve QTS status;
- how to relate knowledge, theory and practice to a course of study;
- self reflection and analysis through personal responses and reading alone;
- developing approaches to sharing views with colleagues and fellow students.

Readers will develop their skills in relating theory to practice through:

- preparatory reading;
- analysis;
- personal responses;
- practical implications and activities;
- further reading.

Primary professional studies

This book will form a core source of reference and reflection for you as you train to teach in the primary sector. It is designed to reflect the key areas of study and development, and thus mirrors the structure of the complementary text *Achieving QTS: Professional Studies: Primary Phase* (Jacques and Hyland, 2003).

The Standards for the award of Qualified Teacher Status (QTS) by the Teacher Training Agency (TTA) have developed since 2002 to include a greater emphasis upon developing professional values and practice. At the core of this set of standards is your ability to reflect and evaluate your own practice and that of others around you.

Key themes focus on:

- the role and voice of learners in their own learning;
- the nature of the curriculum – as delivered content or negotiated process.

This text will provide you with an opportunity to:

- engage with issues at a theoretical level, with reference to key or seminal texts in the field;
- explore the context in which teachers are working, with reference to key historical and legislative developments;
- reflect on your own principles and development as a teacher and consider how this impacts on your work in the classroom.

The book is organised into four sections:

- Section 1: Planning and assessment

- Section 2: Management, organisation and delivery
- Section 3: Children and individual needs
- Section 4: Becoming a professional

Each section is subdivided into a series of short chapters. Each chapter is structured around the key reflective prompts *What? Why?* and *How?* Each of these prompts is explored through a short extract from a key or seminal text in the field. In order to support you in analysing each extract, you will have the opportunity to:

- read a short analysis of the extract;
- provide personal responses;
- consider practical implications.

You will also be shown links to:

- other supporting texts;
- the QTS Standards;
- other sections in this book and in the *Achieving QTS* series.

A note on extracts

Where possible, extracts are reproduced in full but of necessity many have had to be cut. References to other sources embedded within the extracts are not included in this book. Please refer to the extract source for full bibliographical information about any of these.

The author

Sue Kendall-Seatter is currently Head of Primary Education at Canterbury Christ Church University. Having taught in primary schools in south London, she moved into higher education in 1995 where she lectured in primary education at Goldsmiths College. Her curriculum expertise lies in the fields of primary religious education, spiritual development and professional studies. Recent publications include: Kendall, S, *Pilgrimages and Journeys*. Wayland, 2001; Grainger, T and Kendall-Seatter, S, 'Drama and Spirituality: Reflective Connections', *International Journal of Children's Spirituality* 8(1), 2003; Allebone, B, Griffiths, J, Kendall, S, Sidgwick, S, 'The participation of schools in initial teacher education in the London region', in Menter, I, Hutchings, M, Ross, A (eds.) *The Crisis in Teacher Supply: Research and Strategies for Retention*. Stoke-on-Trent: Trentham Books, 2002; Grainger, T and Kendall-Seatter, S (2004) 'Drama and spiritual development' in Dowling, E and Scarlett, G (eds.) *An Encyclopaedia of Spiritual and Religious Development in Childhood and Adolescence*. Thousand Oaks: Sage.

Series editor

Professor Sonia Blandford is Pro-Vice Chancellor (Dean of Education) at Canterbury Christ Church University, one of the largest providers of initial teacher training and professional development in the United Kingdom. Following a successful career as a teacher in primary and secondary schools, Sonia has worked in higher education for nine years. She has acted as an education consultant to ministries of education in Eastern Europe, South America and South Africa and as an adviser to the European Commission, LEAs and schools. She co-leads the Teach First initiative. The author of a range of education management texts, she has a reputation for her straightforward approach to difficult issues. Her publications include: *Middle Management in Schools* (Pearson), *Resource Management in Schools* (Pearson), *Professional Development Manual* (Pearson), *School Discipline Manual* (Pearson), *Managing Special Educational Needs in Schools* (Sage), *Managing Discipline in Schools* (Routledge), *Managing Professional Development in Schools* (Routledge), *Financial Management in Schools* (Optimus), *Remodelling Schools: Workforce Reform* (Pearson) and *Sonia Blandford's Masterclass* (Sage).

Acknowledgements

Every effort has been made to trace the copyright holders and to obtain their permission for the use of copyright material. The publisher and author will gladly receive information enabling them to rectify any error or omission in subsequent editions.

The author and publisher would like to thank the following for permission to reproduce copyright material:

Arthur, J, Davison, J and Lewis M, *Professional Values and Practice*, RoutledgeFalmer 2005. Reproduced with kind permission of Taylor & Francis; Bearne, E (ed), *Differentiation and Diversity*, Routledge 1996. Reproduced with kind permission of Taylor & Francis; Bigger, S and Brown, E (eds), *Spiritual, Moral, Social and Cultural Development,* David Fulton 1999. Reproduced with kind permission of David Fulton Publishers www.fultonpublishers.co.uk; Blandford, S, *School discipline manual*, Pearson Education 2004. Reproduced with kind permission of Pearson Education; Browne, A and Haylock, D, *Professional issues for primary teachers*, Paul Chapman Publishing 2004. Reproduced with kind permission of Sage Publications; Clipson-Boyles, S (ed), *Putting research into practice*, David Fulton 2000. Reproduced with kind permission of David Fulton Publishers www.fultonpublishers.co.uk; Cole, M (ed), *Professional values and practice for teachers and student teachers* 2nd edition, David Fulton 2002. Reproduced with kind permission of David Fulton Publishers www.fultonpublishers.co.uk; Desforges, C (ed), *An Introduction to Teaching: Psychological Perspectives*, Blackwell Publishing 1995; DfES, *Behaviour in the classroom: A course for newly qualified teachers*, DfES 2004. Reproduced with kind permission of DfES/© Crown Copyright; DfES, *Code of practice on the identification and assessment of special needs, Fundamental Principles and Success Factors,* DfES 2001. Reproduced with kind permission of DfES/© Crown Copyright; DfES, *Using the National Healthy School Standard to Raise Boys' Achievment*, DfES 2005. Reproduced with kind permission of DfES; DfES/Macready, C, *Using Data to Narrow the Achievement Gap*, DfES 2005. Reproduced with kind permission of DfES; Erricker, C and Erricker, J, *Reconstructing religious, spiritual and moral education*, RoutledgeFalmer 2000. Reproduced with kind permission of Taylor & Francis; Black,

Personal acknowledgements

My thanks to the Primary Team at Canterbury Christ Church University for critical friendship, professional support and your dedication to the highest standards in primary education. And at home, my thanks to Bob, Sophie and Ellen for your patience, questions and remembering the 'mummy-wine' juice to keep me writing.

Section 1: Planning and assessment

1 Planning and preparation for teaching

By the end of this chapter you should have:

- further considered **why** effective and thorough planning and preparation are key to effective learning and teaching;
- reflected on **what** criteria to consider in order to support effective planning and preparation;
- analysed **how** you plan and prepare, with reference to competing curriculum models.

Linking your learning

- Jacques, K and Hyland, R (2003) *Achieving QTS. Professional studies: primary phase*, Chapter 2. Exeter: Learning Matters.

Professional Standards for QTS
3.1.1–3.1.5

Introduction

Planning and preparing for working in the classroom with a group of learners is the foundation of your career as a teacher. While the nature, scope and format of the planning will change over your career the fact remains that all teachers plan and prepare for the learning of the children they are teaching. The breadth of what is involved is vast and is much more than writing a lesson plan and ensuring all resources are ready. A good teacher will plan and prepare for:

- the children's learning and assessment, including the resources needed;
- other adults involved, or specialist support workers;
- themselves;
- the unexpected.

This list may appear straightforward but it will only be effective if it is informed by your own views on how teaching and learning should operate in a classroom context. This chapter is designed to allow you to reflect upon your own views in an informed manner.

It is the personal responsibility of teachers to ensure that the learning they facilitate is planned. While teachers may work collaboratively to plan a series of lessons, or even team teach, it is important that individual teachers takes ownership for the learning in their classroom or setting. This will not only ensure a higher quality of learning but will assist teachers in managing their own workload. Kyriacou (1991) explores the factors impacting upon teacher stress levels and self-esteem, noting that effective time management is key.

Planning and preparation are also a professional responsibility. As a result of initiatives to remodel the education workforce (*Education Act*, DfES, 2002) and extend the role of schools (DfES, 2004b) all teachers will find themselves working with a range of adults and fellow professionals. It will no longer be the case that individual teachers will be working alone with their class for extended periods. Collaborative planning and preparation are central to the success of these initiatives, and teachers will need to be able to draw on the expertise of fellow adults as well as to share their planning with a wider audience.

Most importantly, planning and preparation can be viewed as a moral responsibility. In Northern Ireland the General Teaching Council sums this up by stating that each new teacher is expected to *like and care for children, and seek to promote the development of the whole child* (Northern Ireland Department for Education, 1999). The ethical response to this value base will be that the class teacher will want to ensure the best possible learning opportunities for the children in his or her care, and thorough and careful planning will facilitate this.

Two fundamental questions underpin the discussion throughout this chapter which you, as a reader, will be guided to explore.

1. Which model of curriculum planning?
2. What is the role of the learner in planning?

Personal response

What do you consider to be the role of the learner in the planning and preparation stage?

Why?

This section aims to encourage you to reflect on why teachers plan by challenging the notion that planning is principally a way of ensuring the optimum delivery method for the selected content. You are asked to consider the learner and the learning as the reasons *why* teachers plan.

Before you read the following extract, read:

www.nc.uk.net/nc_resources/html/valuesAimsPurposes.shtml

This link provides access to the aims, values and purposes of the National Curriculum.

Extract: Dadds, M (2002) 'The 'hurry-along' curriculum', in Pollard, A (ed) *Readings for Reflective Teaching*, 173–175

One major effect of central reforms in primary schools in the past ten years has been an increase in the 'hurry-along curriculum' (Dadds, 1994). 'Coverage' has become a more dominant planning and teaching issue for teachers than learning itself (Pollard *et al.*

1992; Dadds, 1994; Warharn and Dadds, 1998; Pollard and Triggs 2000). The effects of this have been at least twofold.

First, the hurry-along curriculum has diminished the frequency of responsive teaching in which teachers take cues for their pedagogical moves from the responses of children. Under the pressure of curriculum delivery, many have reported moving children too quickly through curriculum material, knowing that understanding suffers in the process (Pollard *et al.*, 1992; Warharn and Dadds, 1998). Even the children themselves 'have a sense of time as a scarce resource' (Triggs and Pollard, 1998, p. 112). This dilemma between coverage and understanding that has been generated in the past ten years, has led to an overemphasis on convergent teaching led by predetermined objectives. There is extensive documentation and debate in the literature of some of the pedagogical consequences of an overemphasis on convergent teaching (for example, Barnes *et al.*, 1969; Hull, 1985; Dadds, 1994; Black and William, 1998). Here I review an illustrative example from a secondary lesson (Barnes *et al.*, 1969) that highlights the nature of the pedagogical problem. In this, we see a teacher's sights set so firmly on the learning objective in the science lesson that he cannot hear the clues the children are giving him about their constructivist learning strategies:

Teacher: You get the white … what we call casein … that's er … protein … which is good for you … it'll help to build bones … and the white is mainly the casein and so it's not actually a solution … it's a suspension of very fine particles together with water and various other things which are dissolved in water …

Pupil: Sir, at my old school I shook my bottle of milk up and when I looked at it again all the side was covered with … er … like particles and … er … could they be the white particles of milk …?

Pupil 2: Yes, and gradually they would sediment out, wouldn't they, to the bottom …?

Pupil 3: When milk goes very sour though it smells like cheese, doesn't it?

Pupil 4: Well, it is cheese, isn't it, if you leave it long enough?

Teacher: Anyway, can we get on? … We'll leave a few questions for later.

In trying to make sense of the new idea, the children try to link it to what is known and familiar in good constructivist fashion. It is to the teacher's credit that he allows the discussion to move around the children, rather than keeping tight control of every response. Yet he misses the opportunity to reinforce the validity of the children's learning strategy by moving towards his objective prematurely. He could, alternatively, have taken a little more time to travel round a learning loop to help the children anchor their thinking more effectively to their previous knowledge. The hurry-along curriculum for information could, thus, have been transformed into a wait-a-while curriculum for reflection and understanding. In the event, however, there is a conflict between a pedagogy for delivery and a pedagogy for learning. Under the pressure of coverage, learning is sacrificed for teaching.

What will be the long-term effects of a hurry-along pedagogy on children's understanding? Does it affect their attitudes towards their learning and towards a sense of their own ability to participate thoughtfully in learning discussions? Evidence on teacher wait-time (Budd-Rowe, 1974; Black and William, 1998) suggests that this may be so. When teachers slow down their response to children's questions and answers, benefits begin to emerge. Children who are slower to respond begin to participate more effectively. Teachers' questions and responses become more thoughtful and more complex, as do the children's. Teachers' concepts of the less able children are transformed as time and space allow these children to offer more of themselves in learning events. The self-esteem of less able children is enhanced through their increased participation (Budd-Rowe, 1974). 'What is essential is that any dialogue should evoke thoughtful reflection in which all pupils can be encouraged to take part' (Black and William, 1998, p. 12). The time created in wait-time pedagogy seems to shift the balance of power in the participation stakes and leads to these improvements in quality teaching and learning.

Yet nothing of these politics of wait-time pedagogy appear in current central initiatives. Indeed, when Black and William published their research early in 1998, it was met with public scorn and derision by aspects of the national press and Her Majesty's Chief Inspector. One cannot help wondering whether the notion of 'pace' and predetermined objectives that are prominent features of the literacy hour pedagogy (DfEE, 1998b) will contribute further to the difficulties of the hurry-along curriculum, encouraging teachers, yet once more, to prioritize coverage over understanding. This is not to say that many children will not benefit from more briskness and pace in teaching and from the clarity that predetermined objectives sometimes bring. But we may need a broader, more complex, debate about whose pace and objectives are appropriate in whole-class teaching contexts. It may also be appropriate to revisit Eisner's (1977) distinction between instructional and expressive objectives, which allows teachers to distinguish between intended and unintended learning outcomes. The current narrow focus on instructional objectives and predetermined outcomes may prevent curriculum designers from seeing as valuable or worthwhile any learning that was not initially intended.

As a second effect, the hurry-along curriculum has minimized the opportunities for teachers to draw children's own interests and questions firmly into curriculum planning and teaching. When central agencies have a strong and heavily loaded sense of what children should be learning then there may be little time to consider what children themselves feel they would be interested to learn (Pollard and Triggs, 2000). Children are fortunate today if their interests map onto the school's rolling curriculum programme for the year. If they do not, those interests may go forever unkindled. In an action research study I supported, the teacher researchers decided to investigate children's views of what would make an interesting curriculum for them. One teacher researcher, working with five- to seven-year-olds, discovered that young children were consistently able to articulate their own interests and the topics that they would like to see represented in the curriculum. Five-year-old Alex, for example, had a clear sense of his own learning interests in the face of his daily directed experiences:

I would like to hav.	I would like to have
a topicke theat is.	a topic that is
birds bicos I like.	birds because I like
birds and bicos.	birds and because
birds ar intresti	birds are interesting

and bicos birds can fly.	and because birds can fly
bicos we crant do maths	because we can't do maths
and riting all the time	and writing all the time

What surprised Alex's teacher was not only that Alex had strong desires that were not being fulfilled, but that he perceived his learning experiences to be dominated so much by 'the basics'. For Alex, mathematics and writing were, the teacher later concluded, taking on the hue of penal servitude. What lessons do children learn about the value and status of their own questions and interests if these are never acknowledged within the curriculum; if they never form the basis for serious learning in schools? What do they learn about the politics of knowledge in these circumstances? Is there a danger that others' knowledge and questions will forever seem to be superior to one's own? Under these conditions, classroom experiences are certainly not leading children 'to develop the skills and attitudes associated with being the kind of lifelong learners that we are told will be characteristic of the next century' (Pollard and Triggs, 2000). This should be warning enough not to continue down this particular pedagogical road, for Alex's experience was not isolated. There is accumulated evidence that that self-directed pupil learning can lead to quality learning outcomes of an astonishing kind, and to high levels of independence in thought and action (for example, Bissex, 1980; Calkins, 1983; Graves, 1983; Dadds, 1986; Fraser, 1987; Drummond, 1993; Hart, 1996). Teachers who have retained the courage to diverge from preset objectives to follow children's interests may have something powerful to offer.

Analysis

During your preparatory reading for this section you will have been reminded that the two aims of the school curriculum are:

- to provide opportunities for all children to learn and to achieve;
- to promote children's spiritual, moral, social and cultural development and prepare all children for the opportunities, responsibilities and experiences of life.

These two aims are achieved through the vehicle of the National Curriculum, which explicitly states that its existence serves to:

- establish an entitlement;
- establish standards;
- promote continuity and coherence;
- promote public understanding.

These are laudable ambitions, yet Dadds (2002) would argue that they have in part contributed to an overemphasis on content and delivery in the classroom. Until 2002, with the introduction of *Qualifying to Teach* (TTA, 2003c), the curriculum for the initial training of teachers had focused on subject knowledge and delivery. This was supported by a plethora of programmes for serving teachers that focused on how to deliver the new strategies for teaching literacy and numeracy.

Dadds identifies two key effects of the 'hurry-along' curriculum:

- a reduction in responsive teaching;
- a diminishing role for the children's own interests in planning.

Practical implications and activities

Working with a peer, describe particular instances in your classroom experience.

1. When you changed the direction or content of a lesson as a result of the responses of the children:

   - What impact did this have on the children?
   - What impact did this have on you as the teacher?

2. When you planned the lesson or series of activities around the interests of the children:

   - How did this influence achievement?
   - How did you ensure you had an accurate understanding of the children's interests?

Take time to revisit 1 and 2 above, this time reflecting on the occasions when you have not changed the lesson in response to the children, or when you have not made explicit reference to the known interests of the children.

More recent developments in policy and practice have signalled the scope for a shift in emphasis in curriculum planning and delivery. In introducing the National Primary Strategy (DfES, 2003b), Charles Clarke, the Secretary of State for Education, notes that:

> Children learn better when they are excited and engaged – but what excites and engages them best is truly excellent teaching which challenges them and shows them what they can do. When there is joy in what they are doing, they learn to love learning. (Clarke, 2003, p3)

Alongside Workforce Reform (DfES, 2002), which provides teachers with more time to plan, and *Every Child Matters* (DfES, 2003c), which places the child at the centre of the process, one could argue that the reason why teachers plan can now be grounded in a constructivist cycle. This is focused on building from where the child is, with informed space for reflection.

What?

This section aims to support you in evaluating the criteria for planning, and in considering *what* it is you should be including or excluding when you come to plan for the learning in your classroom.

Before you read the following extract, read:

- Mortimore, P, Sammons, P, Stoll, L, Lewis, D and Russell, E (1994) 'Teacher Expectations', in Pollard, A and Bourne, J (eds) *Teaching and Learning in the Primary School.* London: Routledge.

This short chapter will prompt you to reflect on how your attitudes, bias and understanding need to be acknowledged as you begin to plan and prepare.

Extract: Tann, S (1995) 'Organizing the Learning Experience', in Desforges, C (ed) *An Introduction to Teaching: Psychological Perspectives*, **pp172-4. Oxford: Blackwell Publishers.**

Criteria for planning

Some psychological theories of learning underline the central need to diagnose, evaluate and meet the child's needs and abilities; utilize and generate motivation in children; offer appropriate rewards and penalties; cast learning in an active mode; give feedback; develop a positive self-concept; plan using a moderate amount of novelty; and recognize the (limited) place of automatic response and rote learning (Morrison and Ridley, 1988, p. 17). The recent changes have highlighted particular dilemmas for teachers as they try to accommodate the new demands and reconcile these with their existing beliefs and principles. These relate to

- the clash between planning and spontaneity
- the question of pupil negotiation and choice
- the need for differentiation and progression.

Planning for spontaneity

The increased attention to planning has required a heightened consciousness of the specific criteria which need to be included in any planning process. This is particularly important when trying to strike a balance between those who believe that a statutory curriculum poses a dichotomy between planning and the spontaneity to be able to respond to individual needs. However, it is perhaps possible to 'plan for spontaneity'. Such a plan could provide a framework of teachers' goals and intentions which is clear enough to help to guide a teacher's decision about flexible adaptations: for example, which spontaneous initiatives it would be advantageous to take into account. After all, a plan is not a blueprint: it merely serves as a guide. Other initiatives from either pupils or teacher, if found to fit in with the overall plan, could therefore be accepted. Initiatives could improve on the original plan and therefore be welcomed. In this way the existence of a plan, the making of which clarifies the teacher's thoughts, allows a teacher to make on-the-spot changes as they reflect-in-action, and it frees them to be spontaneous with confidence.

Planning for negotiated curriculum content

The teacher is responsible for the 'delivery' of a standard curriculum for all pupils. This leads to an increasing emphasis on teacher control of the planning process and outcomes. Nevertheless this does not preclude another feature of the Plowden classroom – the opportunity for pupils to participate in planning their own learning.

This was encouraged in many classrooms as it was believed that it gave ownership of learning to the pupils, and thence responsibility for learning. This in turn enhanced motivation and self-esteem as it increased the likelihood of pupils understanding what they were doing and why, and thus make greater sense of the learning undertaken. The National Curriculum also actively encourages the idea of developing responsibility and learner autonomy by suggesting that pupils share in the critical analysis of their own work and, for example, learn to appraise and improve their technology designs or their story writing. Despite the fact that the National Curriculum has reduced the likelihood of allowing pupils freedom to negotiate the content of their work, it still allows pupils some freedom to negotiate their own preferences and exercise autonomy within prescribed bounds. Hence the need to 'plan for negotiation' should also be a feature of teacher planning.

Planning for negotiated routines

Instead of negotiating content, there are also opportunities for pupils to make decisions regarding 'routines' relating to the ordering and duration of tasks. For example, pupils can be set tasks for the day or week, and they decide in which order tasks will be completed. Having made their choices, the teacher may only remind them when to move on to the next task. This may be at a given 'all change' signal (which can alleviate pressure on any resource area and ensure that pupils are distributed safely around the classroom). Some teachers allow pupils to decide whether to do a little of each subject daily or in large blocks of concentrated time. The pupils are therefore free to choose when they change. Such a system is often combined with the additional responsibility for the pupils to mark their own work using the 'Teacher's answer book', for example for regular computational exercises in maths, cloze exercises in English or multiple choice checks in other subjects.

Planning for differentiation

Although the curriculum entitles all children to common, standardized content it is also necessary to match the curriculum to meet individual needs in terms of levels of achievement. This requires a considerable amount of differentiation. This is typically achieved in a number of ways. Teachers can plan the same task for every pupil and expect differentiation in terms of the quality and quantity of output. Or differentiation can occur through varied input achieved by the teacher's adaptation of the task to suit different pupils' abilities. Or differentiation can be directed at the support stage: after giving the same task to all pupils, the teacher can plan more help to particular groups or individuals as is appropriate in order to help them to understand and complete the task and thereby experience success. Hence 'planning for differentiation' is also an important component of teacher planning.

Planning for progression

This can include moving from simple to complex concepts, basic primary to derived secondary ones, from concrete to abstract ones. Tasks and materials, too, are important: from closed (right/wrong) to open (interpretative/imaginative) tasks, from first-hand to secondary resources, artefacts to information books. The demands of the social context should also be considered.

Analysis

It may be tempting, when faced with a class of children to teach, to launch into the content of what you are going to deliver. The National Curriculum, National Strategy documents, and the school's interpretation of these, will provide you with much of this detail. Your preparatory reading for this section will have alerted you to the many additional factors related to your knowledge and understanding of the children and your relationships with them that will have a profound impact on the learning that takes place. Mortimore et al. (1994) categorise these as:

- age differences;
- social class differences;
- sex differences;
- ethnic differences;
- ability differences;
- behaviour differences.

As a teacher and as an individual you will have a different interpretation and understanding of the opportunities and issues such differences present. While it is expected good practice that teachers will differentiate according to need it is imperative that you, as an individual, acknowledge your preconceptions at the planning stage.

Tann's (1995) criteria for planning suggest a way forward to ensure that planning remains responsive even during delivery.

Practical implications and activities

1. Select a lesson or session plan that you have taught. Colour code those elements of the plan and evaluation that are linked to:

- practical learning organisation;
- pedagogical learning interaction.

2. Could you rework the plan to include provision for:

- spontaneity?
- negotiated curriculum content?

Tann (1995) highlights the tensions and dilemmas that may arise as a consequence of the desire to remain responsive throughout the planning, preparation and delivery stage. Arthur, Davison and Lewis (2005) would suggest that this tension arises from teachers focusing their reflective energies on the technical elements of their practice. The curriculum they are required to teach has been conceptualised in terms of knowledge content and thus *successful teaching is simply teaching that brings about the desired learning in narrow subject terms* (p7). Tickle's (1996) research implies that for evaluation to be meaningful it must have a basis in the values of education. It would follow that these will be grounded in the relationships between, and with, learner and teacher, and would thus support an emphasis on planning for the *pedagogical learning interactions* (Tann, 1995). The changing emphasis in recent education policy and legislation seems to lend support to a focus on *communication between teacher and pupil* (Tann, 1995, p174) as being at the heart of effective planning and preparation.

How?

This section explores the different historical and contemporary views that have influenced *how* the curriculum is structured and planned. It challenges you to consider planning to facilitate the development of key skills that are transformative.

Before you read the following extract, read:

- DfES (2004a) *Learning and Teaching in the Primary Years. Professional Development Resources.*

These are professional development materials to support planning in primary schools. Parts 1 and 2 are particularly useful when considering planning models.

Extract: Pollard, A and Tann, S (1993*) Reflective Teaching in the Primary School***, 2nd edition, pages 132(1.1)–134. London: Cassell.**

Primary practice
Historically, there have been two major alternative strategies for curricular planning within primary schools: focusing on separate subjects or planning forms of integration between subjects. The strengths of subject teaching, in terms of curricular progression, are also its weakness regarding overall coherence in pupil learning experiences. Unfortunately, the reverse is also true, in that the coherence of integrated work can lead to fragmentation in the understanding of particular subjects.

While subject-based approaches were common in what Blyth (1965) called the 'preparatory school tradition', integrated approaches, using 'topics', have been very significant in primary education ever since the Plowden Report of 1967 (CACE, 1967). Indeed, some would argue that topic work became a distinctive feature of the primary-school ideology. However, the apparent distinctiveness of these approaches conceals a considerable overlap in actual practice.

1.1 The 'basics' and the 'other' curriculum
Whatever is said about the primary curriculum, the evidence from research (e.g. Pollard *et al.*, 1994) and from the prescriptive literature shows that a 'two-curriculum syndrome' is in operation. This argument was powerfully made by Alexander (1984) and reinforced by his later work (Alexander *et al.*, 1989; Alexander, 1992). The two curricula that he had in mind are those of the 'basics' (reading, writing and mathematics) and those of the rest – the 'other' curriculum. Alexander argued that the rhetoric of child-centred education, which is associated with an integrated form of curriculum organization, has prevented teachers from facing the fact that the basics in the curriculum have usually been taught in a relatively discrete and almost subject- based way. It is only with regard to other, less central, areas of the curriculum that attempts to establish integration have really been made. Figure 7.1 shows Alexander's analysis of the major dimensions of the 'two curricula'. Some of the concepts in this model are sophisticated and it will be worth revisiting having read other parts of this chapter.

Alexander's model provides both challenges and insights when considering the curriculum. In particular, it shows how actual primary practice often reflects the pragmatism and judgement of 'what works'. The result is something of a necessary compromise, despite the impression which might sometimes be given by rhetoric from either quarter.

1.2 A subject-based curriculum?

A subject-based curriculum is one which maintains high subject boundaries and thus maintains distinctions between subjects. The resulting curriculum, therefore, is a collection of separate subjects: indeed, it has been called a 'collection curriculum' (Bernstein, 1971). Progression within each separate subject may be strong, though coherence across subjects is likely to be weak.

A philosophical rationale for a subject-based curriculum is that each element is based on logical structures of knowledge which are believed to be unique to that subject or 'form of knowledge' (Hirst and Peters, 1970). Indeed, Alexander *et al.* (1992, p. 17) claimed that subjects are 'some of the most powerful tools for making sense of the world which human beings have ever devised'.

However, the approach is one that primarily appeals to traditionalists. Indeed, perhaps the origin of curriculum subjects can be found in the high status which is attributed to the formal, classical education of public and grammar schools and to a belief that this is the only approach which will deliver competencies in basic subjects (Lawlor, 1988).

Justification/ideology

Social relevance ———	Self-actualization
Societal ———	Individual
Utilitarian ———	Child-centred

View of knowledge

Received ———	Reflexive
Rationalist ———	Empiricist
Positive ———	Negative, anti-knowledge

Organizational characteristics

Subject differentiation ———	Undifferentiated
Extensive codification of knowledge ——— and skills	Little or no codification
Explicit progression of knowledge ——— and skills	Little or no explicit progression

Evaluation

Pre-ordinate/'objective' ———	Responsive/'subjective'

Pedagogy

Teacher-directed ———	Child-initiated

Outcome

Progressive acquisition of knowledge ——— and skills	Learning experiences random and circular
High level of 'match' between ——— learning experiences and child's abilities	Low level of match

Professional training and resources

High priority in initial training ———	Low priority in initial training
Well-developed teacher technology ——— of schemes and materials	Limited teacher technology
Relatively high INSET commitment by ——— teachers and LEAs	Relatively low INSET commitment by teachers and LEAs

Figure 7.1 Dimensions for analysing the primary curriculum
(from Alexander (1984), p. 76)

1.3 An integrated curriculum?

An integrated curriculum is one which draws on several subjects to construct a holistic and, it is hoped, meaningful focus for study (Hunter and Scheirer, 1988).

Many different types of arguments for the desirability of an integrated curriculum have been offered. One suggests that the curriculum should draw on pupil experiences if effective learning is to take place. It is thus considered that the imposition of artificial subject boundaries may inhibit children's understanding.

Another argument is that, in a fast-moving world, new 'subjects' have emerged. These are inter-disciplinary and conceptually linked (Pring, 1976), for instance, environmental studies and media studies. Such issues cross 'forms of knowledge'. For example, aspects of health education require us to make responses which are social, moral and economic as well as scientific. This form of integration was highlighted in some Schools Council projects, such as Place, Time and Society (Blyth, 1975), and even in the modern, subject-based, National Curriculum of England and Wales, it remains in the emphasis on cross-curricular themes (see section 2.2 of this chapter).

A third argument that underpins integrated curricular planning is that a higher priority can be given to generally applicable processes, skills and attitudes if the emphasis on particular subject knowledge is lessened. The idea here is that knowledge is changing so fast in the world that it is more important for children to learn transferable skills than to concentrate on facts which may rapidly become outdated.

Analysis

Recent policy initiatives, such as *Excellence and Enjoyment: The Primary Strategy* (DfES, 2003b), have once again ignited the debates about the nature of the primary curriculum. The support materials for this initiative are extensive and promote a view that there are three *different levels of planning*:

- curriculum mapping and long-term planning;
- medium-term plans;
- short-term plans.
  (DfES, 2004a, p23)

Personal response

Reflect on your personal learning. How do you learn best?

- When information is presented in discrete subject blocks?
- When material is presented in a cross-curricular way?
- When you have control over the content and direction of the learning?
- When you are presented with new and unfamiliar material?
- Or does it vary?

Practical implications and activities

Select a complete set of planning materials from one of your placement schools; this should include all three levels from long-term through to the actual lesson or session plan. You should have been involved in teaching an element of this work.

1. Using Pollard and Tann's (1993) categories for structuring the curriculum, is there an emphasis on:

   - the *basics* and the *other* curriculum?
   - a subject-based curriculum?
   - an integrated curriculum?

2. Can you identify where you feel most comfortable as a teacher? And could you amend the planning to suit your preferred curriculum planning model?

3. Does your preferred method of planning link to your own preferred ways of learning as identified in the response box above?

Pollard and Tann (1993) explore the debates surrounding a subject-based versus an integrated curriculum, which may not be as polarised and exclusive as they are sometimes depicted. Implicit in their discussion is the reality that teachers are skilled in making pragmatic and effective decisions that are responsive to the current learning situation. These decisions are increasingly informed by an analysis of what will be most useful in supporting individual learners to link their learning to previous experiences and interests.

Contemporary writers in the field, such as Hayes (2004), draw attention to the importance of *learning to learn*. The focus here is on equipping the learner with a set of skills and aptitudes that allows them to access, interpret and apply their knowledge and understanding in the curriculum. It could be argued that children have not learnt something until they are able to employ their new-found knowledge and concepts.

If *learning to learn* becomes the principal driving factor behind curriculum design, then the debate between the basics, subject-based or integrated curriculum begins to take on a different perspective. The principal decisions then revolve around which key skills and aptitudes are worthy of promotion and development, and these in turn become the focus of planning.

This is not a new discussion: guidance documentation supporting the implementation of the National Curriculum identified the key skills that should underpin teaching and learning. Currently these skills are:

- communication;
- application of number;
- information technology;
- working with others;
- improving own learning and performance;
- problem-solving;
- information-processing;
- reasoning;

- enquiry;
- creative thinking;
- evaluation.
  (QCA, 1998)

The impetus to focus on the *how* of learning rather than the *what* has been invigorated by an active movement to promote *thinking skills* in primary schools. Much of this work is based on the theories of Gardner and Claxton. Although they themselves express disquiet at what they perceive as the *trivialisation* (Gardner, 1997) and *outrageously misinterpreted* application (Claxton, 1997) of the theories, this has served to raise the profile of the skills and processes of learning.

This draws us back to one of the key themes of this chapter concerning the role of the individual learners and their impact upon the planning and preparation process. It has been suggested that planning decisions need to be informed first by the learning skills needs of the learners and, second, by the knowledge and understanding requirements of the prescribed curriculum. Hayes (2004) talks about learning as transformation and, as such:

> the teacher's role in the [planning] process is to provide the resources, guidance and wisdom that facilitate the learning. Such teaching [and planning] recognises that learning does not consist merely of the linear transfer of an adult's superior intellect to a less knowledgeable pupil but rather an accommodation of the fresh understanding into the child's conceptual framework. (p121)

Summary

This chapter will have supported you in reflecting on the reasons for, nature of and complexities surrounding the planning and preparation process. Your training establishment will be providing you with sample proformas and setting the required expectations for the amount and layers of planning expected as you progress towards achieving QTS. Your placement school will have its own expectations of the teaching staff as to what format and detail is expected when planning for the learning. Often there will be a substantial gap between the expectations of these two institutions regarding you, the trainee teacher. At its best, this can result in a rich professional dialogue about the principles of planning; at worst, it can cause friction about competing expectations. As a trainee teacher, it is important that you are prepared and flexible in all contexts. Having engaged with the issues discussed in this chapter and reflected on your own personal philosophy underpinning the nature and purpose of planning, you will be better placed to learn from and reflect on the differences you will undoubtedly encounter.

Further reading

Arthur, J, Davison, J and Lewis, M (2005) *Professional values and practice: Achieving the Standards for QTS*. London: RoutledgeFalmer.

Hayes, D (2004) *Foundations of primary teaching*, 3rd edition. London: David Fulton.

Hughes, P (2002) *Principles of primary education*, 2nd edition. London: David Fulton.

Kyriacou, C (1991) *Essential teaching skills*. Cheltenham: StanleyThornes.

2 Planning for all abilities: differentiation

By the end of this chapter you should have:

- further considered **why** effective and thorough differentiation is key to ensuring curriculum entitlement for all;
- reflected on **what** criteria to consider in order to support effective differentiation;
- analysed **how** your own developing principles and values of education inform the kind of differentiated curriculum you choose to operate.

Linking your learning

- Jacques, K and Hyland, R (2003) *Achieving QTS. Professional studies: primary phase*, Chapter 3. Exeter: Learning Matters.

Professional Standards for QTS
3.1.1–3.1.3, 3.2.4, 3.3.4, 3.3.6

Introduction

Differentiating the learning you are planning and delivering will allow greater access and achievement for the children you are working with. One could argue that this is the moral and professional responsibility of all teachers, and it certainly supports the National Curriculum's purpose of establishing an entitlement to learning. However, as you might predict, something that sounds simple and straightforward in practice is anything but. Neither is it without controversy and debate. Bearne (1996, p2) hints at this tension by asking:

> does differentiation imply an attempt to identify and widen differences between individual pupils or does it carry with it the notion of welcoming difference while providing equitable access to education for all?

Personal response

What is the link between inclusion, diversity and differentiation? Are they complementary or are they in competition with one another?

The principle underpinning this chapter is that *all* children are individuals, with preferred learning styles, strengths and challenges in their learning. Necessarily, differentiating the learning will cause the teacher to reflect upon each child. The challenge is to explore management strategies that facilitate such a way of working. To this end this chapter will ask you to explore and reflect upon models and layers of differentiation within the context of your own developing views about the nature of the curriculum.

The links with the themes discussed in Chapter 1 will become evident. However, throughout this chapter you are asked to reflect upon two questions.

- What is the role of learners in differentiating their learning?
- What type of relationship do you want to have with the children you are teaching?

Why?

This section aims to encourage you to reflect on *why* teachers plan for differentiated learning, by challenging the notion that the *product* is the principal way of assessing the impact of teaching. You are asked to consider the process of learning as a key factor in determining differentiation.

Before you read the following extract, read:

- Hayes, D (2004) (3rd edn) *Foundations of Primary Teaching*, Part Two: Learning and Teaching.

Although an extract from the above book is included in our Chapter 5, reading the whole of Part Two will provide you with a useful philosophical overview.

Extract: McNamara, S and Moreton, G (1997) *Understanding Differentiation*, pp3–6. London: David Fulton.

When considering the current polarised debate in education about whole class teaching or individual work, setting and streaming or mixed ability, and thinking about the way in which we usually teach, the authors envisaged a model to summarise their approach. They saw the debate and their own approach in the shape of a pair of scales with the arguments of the two polarised sides on either side and their way in the middle. This is outlined in Figure 1.1.

The two sides

Progressive approaches (usually associated with child-centred learning.)	*Traditional approaches*
Mixed ability, mixed groups – this usually means that children are seated in mixed ability groups around tables.	Setting and streaming – grouping by ability.
Individual needs: children's individual needs are the focus, there is an expectation therefore that children will work at different rates, and produce work of different types and varying quality.	Children must be treated the same and equally, no allowances must be made, there are clear criteria and standards. In some European countries this means that children who fail simply repeat a year.

Children's prior experiences are the starting point for a lesson. This sometimes means that the curriculum is built around children's perceived needs, interests and environment. Topic work was an example of this.

The curriculum content is the starting point.
The focus is on knowledge that has been prioritised and which all children need to experience.

Differentiation by outcome, where different standards of work are expected from children of different abilities.

Differentiation by task – teachers try to match the task to the ability of the child.

Differentiation by resource. Teachers set up activities in the room and try to 'extend' them by having conversations with the most able, and provide 'security' by explanations for the least able. This creates a need for more adults in the classroom.

Teachers have usually already sorted children into ability groups and may feel that there is no reason to differentiate further. Those who do prepare worksheets and different types of work for different abilities use text access techniques to help those with literacy difficulties. This is time consuming.

Relaxed informal atmosphere where children are happy and encouraged to talk but talk will be on-task to teacher and off-task to peers. High achieving children will be interested but not stretched or challenged.

Tight formal structures, children not encouraged to talk. Strict routines, much whole class instruction and teaching. No talk for exploration or deeper understanding. Surface Learning the 'norm'. In these circumstances talk is likely to be off-task.

Low expectations usually result from the Differentiation by Outcome.

Low standards and 'refusal' or alienation can develop in children who are constantly given the 'easy' sheet or activity in Differentiation by Task.

Dependency and Learned Helplessness develop because the children are dependent on the teacher for inspiration, organisation of classroom activities and assessment feedback.

Learned Helplessness, negative self-belief and low self-esteem are the negative by-products for the children who are in the low ability group or who receive the low ability work. In our experience once children believe they are no good they cannot perform very well and are unable to do the work even if it is carefully matched to their ability level. Refusal to start 'the work' unless an adult helps them or nags them to write the date, draw a margin, write the question are examples of Learned Helplessness. (1978)

For both sets of teachers, those on the right and those on the left, variety and differences between children both in terms of ability and learning styles are seen as problems, usually to be resolved by 'extra resources.'

It is the authors' experience that children from both ends of the ability range can demonstrate enormous gains in learning if the material is presented in a different way. This happens when children see themselves as being equal in a classroom where difference is encouraged and valued rather than considered abnormal and a cause of extra work for everyone; and when self-belief is positive.

This other way sees variety and difference as an asset. It looks at children's differences and sees them as interesting forms of potential collaboration, with children providing complementary skills for one another. The resourcing issue is then a straightforward one of class size rather than resources for difference in ability.

The model for differentiation
Differentiation is about giving access and entitlement. It should also lead to an end to dependency. A variety of abilities should be seen as an asset and not a problem. The Model for Differentiation is a model based on collaboration between children with different styles and strengths and not on a hierarchy of abilities. Talk is the basis for differentiation, not tasks.

In our model for differentiation where talk and collaboration are the key, the teacher:

- structures learning and assessment so that children can learn through talk as well as reading and writing (Differentiation by Classroom Organisation).
- encourages the children to demonstrate their learning through any media they like, hence offering a variety of recording mechanisms (Differentiation by Outcome, Product).
- teaches children to help each other to set and reach targets and teach each other to improve their work through carefully structured peer tutoring (Differentiation by Paired Task).

This model sees an end to matching tasks to children and a beginning of children deciding for themselves what they need to achieve. This means that children are not repeating work that they can already do which is often an unfortunate consequence of focusing on the 'basics.'

It is through the separation of the learning and assessment that differentiation in this way becomes possible. This method frees up the recording during the learning and enables the child to record in any way they wish – any way that helps them to demonstrate what it is that they can do. It gets formal reading and writing, in the way that is required for assessment purposes, out of the way during the learning process, and paradoxically this has the effect of increasing the amount of reading and writing that goes on in the lesson. This kind of reading and writing is incidental, purposeful and targeted. The amount of spontaneous learning increases enormously.

5. *Revision*. This reactivates ideas/procedures/skills which have not been used for some time.

The study found that 60 per cent of tasks set in Language and Maths were intended as short-term practice, 25 per cent were 'incremental', 6 per cent were enrichment, 6 per cent were intended as long-term revision and only 1 per cent were intended as restructuring.

Pollard's work has clear space and outlets for the learner's voice, with the implication being that the teacher will closely observe and monitor; this will necessarily include listening. It is interesting to read Pollard's work alongside the guidance produced by OFSTED for its inspectors evaluating primary practice. There, too, one can find an emphasis on listening to the learner, but there is a tension here between what Pollard believes is effective task differentiation management and the view conveyed by the inspectorate. Pollard (1997, p200) argues that:

> a reflective teacher needs to monitor closely to try to ensure the best balance between boredom with too easy tasks, frustration with tasks that are too hard, comfort from consolidation tasks and excitement from a task that is challenging but not too daunting.

OFSTED (2003a, Section 4), on the other hand, suggests that its inspectors should:

> probe what pupils know, understand and can do and set this against the expectations of teachers. Any discrepancies give us a clue that not enough is being asked.

While at one level this apparent disagreement relates to what it is reasonable to ask a learner to do in the classroom, it does point to issues around teachers' perceptions of task matching. Pollard's *four stages of analysis* provide a valuable tool for evaluating the appropriateness of tasks to individual learners. Their value lies in the fact that teachers are required to engage actively with their learners, rather than following a more *teacher distant* model suggested at the start of this section.

Practical activities and implications

Using the five types of task demand, below, from Bennett, Desforges, Cockburn, and Wilkinson (1984), can you evaluate a series of lessons you have observed or taught? Select an individual or group and consider how far the tasks set were:

- incremental;
- restructuring;
- enrichment;
- practice;
- revision.

The extract from Pollard (1997) is perhaps alarming in that he highlights so many permutations that might disguise a mismatch of task to learner (or learner to task). However I would suggest that the tool from Bennett et al. (1984), if applied in a manner that assists learners in commenting on their *experience* of the task, would help teachers to build up an accurate picture of the effectiveness of the match.

And as for the OFSTED inspector's question about challenge? If a teacher can confidently explain the fact that s/he has planned for a range of activities that will allow each learner to work through from the *incremental* to the *revision*, with a balance that reflects need, surely there can be no criticism?

How?

This section explores the *how* of differentiation, when set in the context of trying to achieve a curriculum entitlement for all. In order to achieve this you are challenged to explore your own values in relation to equality of opportunity and entitlement.

Personal response

The curriculum which most successfully caters for diversity through differentiation has to accommodate two apparently contradictory requirements – of equity and of individual growth. (Bearne, 1996, p257)

Is this possible? How?

Before you read the following extract, read:

- DfES (2004a) *Learning and Teaching in the Primary Years.* (Professional Development Resources).

Pay particular attention to Part 3, Planning for Inclusion, p39 and *the three principles of inclusion.*

Extract: Doddington, C (1996) 'Grounds for differentiation. Some values and principles in primary education considered', in Bearne, E (ed) *Differentiation and diversity*, pages 38–39. London: Routledge.

The idea of differentiation seems to invite a focus on the differences between people rather than what is common. This may seem at first to be a straightforward idea. It is not quite so uncomplicated, however, since the degree to which we consider the human race as comprising individuals with differences, or as a mass of humanity with much in common, can vary. Sensitivity to the extent of 'difference' between people has grown as the idea of the individual has increased in significance. Also, difference between people is discerned not so much by simple identification, but through the values and purposes that are held in mind. For this reason, alerting ourselves to difference is seen as appropriate at some times and irrelevant at others. This means that, depending on the context, any perceived difference, such as race, gender or age, may be acknowledged and influential or deliberately disregarded. Educational contexts are good examples of such contrasting approaches where particular values and priorities can exert pressure to distinguish between people, or alternatively, disregard difference in favour of common provision. Any claim in schools for differentiation or common entitlement then, rests less on empirical evidence, more on values, assumptions and professional judgement. In this chapter I will examine some of the underlying assumptions of commonality and difference in education and explore some of the values and priorities on which those conceptions are based. I then go on to look at ways in which apparently contrasting positions can be drawn together in carefully conceived classroom practice.

There seem to be oppositions in educational thinking between views which concentrate on the individual and those which look at common features or qualities. Many studies of learning encourage teachers to consider awareness of personality, background and experience, cultural influence and the subtle effects of myriad social encounters on people. At the same time there has been a continued debate about what should be seen in education as common provision for all. This apparent tension echoes a wider debate between those who wish to promote individualism and those who search for what connects humanity or particular groups. Despite the controversy, this dichotomy may be misleading when we think about the classroom context. For example, differentiation in the classroom may require us to focus on individuals and difference by making distinctions between children's performance in a particular task. However, it is also related to what should be common, since the principle of entitlement is to provide equal access to what is deemed of value and essential for all. Differentiation may be required precisely to achieve that access. Any structure put forward as the basis for a curriculum will rest in part on judgements made about value and emphasis and in part on individuals and entitlement. The teacher in the primary classroom therefore consciously, or subconsciously, expresses her values and priorities when she determines what will be common experiences for all and what learning experiences are designed to be different for different children.

Analysis

It seems the key question raised by Doddington is about the extent to which you, as a teacher, perceive the children you are teaching as individuals first and foremost, or as a group displaying differences. Is it ethically justifiable to seek out the differences in order to treat differently? By and large it seems that the moral imperative to provide access to a curriculum entitlement outweighs the resulting need to look for difference. As Arthur, Davison and Lewis note, *'differentiation' in the classroom is a current term within education discourse that has very positive connotations* (2005, p55).

Thus, if we need to seek out difference, how do we do it in an informed and sensitive manner? Government guidance (DfES, 1999) suggests that teachers need to take account of *boys and girls, pupils with special educational needs, pupils with disabilities, pupils from all social and cultural backgrounds and pupils from different ethnic groups.* Arthur, Davison and Lewis (2005, p53) provide a more comprehensive list and add:

- pupils from particular faith communities;
- travellers;
- asylum seekers;
- refugees;
- working-class children;
- middle-class children;
- pupils with English as an additional language;
- gifted and talented pupils;
- disabled pupils;
- children in the care of the local authority;
- any pupil at risk of disaffection or exclusion.

This list of categories serves to highlight a range of factors that will impact upon the ability of children to access the learning and, therefore, could well justify modification of planning and/or delivery of the curriculum. While it is imperative that teachers make every attempt to be informed about the background, culture and needs of each child it would be a dangerous assumption to make that this list is exhaustive or that all children included in it require the same level or type of differentiation.

Practical implications and activities

1. Identify a lesson or activity you have taught or observed. Think about:

   - learning objectives;
   - teaching styles;
   - access.
     (DfES, 2004a)

2. How would you differentiate the curriculum in order to facilitate the learning for an identified group or individual?

3. Why did you choose this element of the curriculum?

4. What expertise or knowledge do you have about the learning needs of the individual or group?

In seeking to differentiate the curriculum, according to Doddington (1996), teachers are intuitively overlaying their own value system on the learning. In making decisions about what knowledge, concepts or skills are to be included or excluded in order to differentiate, the teacher is deciding what part of the curriculum will be available to all and which will be different.

Summary

I began this chapter by commenting upon the apparently uncontested and straightforward assumption that differentiation of the curriculum is a good thing. During your training you will be asked by those observing you as you teach to *tell me how you ensured all children could achieve in that lesson?* What they want to see on your lesson plan is a range of different tasks, or targeted support, or your expected outcomes from varying groups in your classroom. You will observe experienced and skilled teachers at work, where differentiation is woven through all that is happening in the room. This chapter will have raised questions in your mind.

- Am I right to amend the curriculum content for those with a specific need? Or am I denying them access to experiences open to others?
- How do I ensure that my tasks are differentiated in such a way as to stretch, consolidate and enrich the learning for all the children? Are some learners just biding their time while, for others, all learning tasks present them with frustration and failure?
- Am I delivering the content in my way or am I listening to the children for clues and cues to direct the differentiation?

Further reading

Cole, M (ed) (2002) *Professional Values and Practice for Teachers and Student Teachers*, 2nd Edition. London: David Fulton.

Desforges, C (ed) (1995) *An Introduction to Teaching.* Oxford: Blackwell.

Pollard, A (ed) (2002) *Readings for Reflective Teaching*. London: Continuum.

3 Assessment, recording and reporting on children's work

By the end of this chapter you should have:

- further considered **why** assessment, monitoring, recording and reporting are important factors in contributing to the enhancement of children's performance;
- critically evaluated **what** criteria to consider in order to support effective assessment, recording and reporting;
- analysed **how** your own developing principles and values of education inform the kind of assessment you deploy and how you use assessment data that is reported locally and centrally.

Linking your learning

- Jacques, K and Hyland, R (2003) *Achieving QTS. Professional studies: primary phase*, Chapter 4. Exeter: Learning Matters.

Professional Standards for QTS
3.2.1–3.2.7

Introduction

The first two chapters in this section considered the preparation and presentation of the work you plan for your children. This chapter explores the impact. Assessment and recording are politically sensitive and controversial issues in the world of education. The push to raise standards was high on the agenda of the Conservative and then Labour governments in the 1980s and 1990s, and was a driving force behind the introduction of the National Curriculum. This led to the introduction of a raft of external and centrally determined testing mechanisms. League and performance tables were the inevitable outcome. For many teachers, assessment became divorced from their daily planning and teaching. In the late 1990s the Assessment Reform Group was charged with redressing the balance and exploring the use of *assessment for learning*. The impetus and principles underpinning this project are supported throughout this chapter.

Personal response

Reflect on an aspect of your own learning when considering these prompts:

I am learning to ...

I will know I have achieved this because ...
(adapted from a model by Shirley Clarke, 2001)

Note down your responses. Share them with a trusted colleague.

- What is common?
- Where do the differences lie?
- Why?

Links with the themes discussed in Chapters 1 and 2 will continue to emerge. However, throughout this chapter you are asked to reflect on two questions.

- What is the role of the learner in the assessment process?
- Who owns and uses the information you gather through the assessment process?

Why?

The aim of this section is to encourage you to reflect on *why* teachers are required to engage in assessment, recording and reporting. You are asked to reflect on the role of the learner in the assessment process.

Before you read the following extract, read:

- Pollard, A (2002) *Reflective Teaching*, 2nd Edition. Chapter 14, 'Assessment. How are we monitoring learning and performance?'. London: Continuum.

This provides an analytical overview of the key issues.

Extract: Headington, R (2003) *Monitoring, Assessment, Recording, Reporting and Accountability: Meeting the Standards*, **2nd edition, pp110–113. London: David Fulton.**

MARRA is a linchpin within this array of standards. It is a combination of interrelated assessment issues, all of which have a direct relationship with pupils' learning. MARRA requires a critical awareness of the theory upon which assessment practice is based. It requires the ability to operate effectively at many different levels, from close diagnostic work with an individual pupil to recognising how targets are used to improve national results in literacy and numeracy. It requires the ability to work with a range of personnel, from pupils and LSAs to governors and parents. It requires a recognition of the roles and responsibilities of others within the education system, from the school senior management team to the Secretary of State for Education. It requires an awareness of the importance of MARRA to people at different levels of the education system, including politicians and policy makers, LEAs and schools, parents and teachers. It requires the ability to use assessment to improve the quality of teaching and an understanding of the centrality of pupils in the assessment process.

7.2 Why is MARRA important to politicians and policy makers?
Politicians and policy makers have had a considerable impact upon MARRA since the 1980s. A plethora of education legislation and guidance has brought into being centralised systems and structures, regulations and responsibilities. Vast sums of money have been spent putting legislation and guidance into action. Legislation has focused

upon curriculum content and its assessment. It has required open access to information about pupils' performance and has enhanced parents' rights. Guidance has helped teachers to interpret the published curriculum and recognise the requirements of associated statutory assessment. It has recommended lesson structures in the key areas of literacy and numeracy and planning frameworks in other curriculum areas. Together legislation and guidance have informed teachers of what they must teach, recommended how it should be taught and have enabled these areas to be monitored nationally through statutory assessment and inspection.

Technology has aided the collection, interrogation and dissemination of data from statutory assessment. Politicians and policy makers use the data, based increasingly upon the specific and measurable areas of reading, writing and number, to evaluate the quality of education available and to make comparisons with other countries. Successive governments have looked to models from business and industry to determine how 'higher standards' can be achieved in education. By deciding where and how to spend financial resources, governments have highlighted the areas of education which they considered to be most important. For example, national targets and a greater emphasis upon literacy and numeracy through national strategy initiatives, along with booster classes for more able pupils, summer schools for those who need time to 'catch up' with their peers and homework for all, followed research and international comparison which suggested that levels of literacy and numeracy were insufficient (OFSTED 1996b; Reynolds and Farrell 1996).

Government spending on resources and initiatives is evaluated in terms of its value for money and provides politicians and policy makers with accountability evidence, demonstrating the effectiveness of their strategies to the taxpayers who ultimately pay for the education service.

7.3 Why is MARRA important to LEAs and schools?
LEAs and schools work together to manage government resources and initiatives in practice. They use MARRA to determine how financial and practical resources should be allocated to benefit pupils and schools. Results of summative statutory assessments are used to monitor trends and inconsistencies and to target areas of need.

LEA advisory and inspection services work with schools to develop and implement OFSTED action plans and School Development Plans. For example, if in-service training is required upon specific aspects of curriculum, such as mental mathematics, LEA advisory staff may work in the school, with some or all members of staff, or they may run LEA courses to address particular needs. Similarly LEA specialists work with ENCOs to devise and implement statements of special educational need for individual pupils, and they support additional provision for pupils with EAL and those who are gifted and talented.

LEAs often run training courses for teachers in statutory assessment and related areas of professional development such as transfer, moderation and involving pupils in self-assessment. LEA personnel are involved in audits during the statutory assessment period, checking that administration arrangements have been carried out satisfactorily and processing optical mark reader sheets at Key Stage 1. They may be invited into schools to explain elements of the statutory assessment process and the use of comparative results, to staff or to parents.

Schools use statutory assessment results to monitor the progress of groups and individual pupils. They compare the results of their own school with others of a similar nature, to determine whether the school targets they have set are realistic and challenging. They monitor the progress of groups of pupils and subject areas to determine whether different approaches to teaching and learning, such as setting by ability in mathematics, may be more effective. They use cumulative data to track and predict the progress of individual pupils, target their learning needs and provide appropriate support.

Schools also keep parents informed of the progress of their own children in relation to the age group within the school and nationally. They work with parents to explore and monitor contributory factors, including the social, physical and emotional, which may affect a pupil's academic progress, seeking the assistance of outside agencies such as Social Services where necessary.

7.4 Why is MARRA important to parents and teachers?
Parents and teachers use MARRA to ensure the progress of individual pupils. Parents can monitor the progress of their children in relation to previous past performance in the Foundation Stage Profile and End of Key Stage tests. They can use the criteria of the National Curriculum document to identify what their children know, do and understand in relation to the levels of attainment. They can compare their children with the performance of other children of the same age at the school and with others of the same age nationally. They can discuss their children's progress with the class teacher and, with her and the children, determine appropriate targets and how they can help in the learning process.

MARRA encourages teachers to monitor and assess the learning and learning needs of all the pupils in a class as a complementary part of the planning and assessment cycles. The processes of recording and reporting ensure regular and objective approaches are developed and maintained and these in turn enable accountability to pupils, parents and professionals. Teachers use formative and diagnostic assessment to make the work undertaken with pupils more appropriate to their learning needs. They use summative assessments to bring together many aspects of pupils' learning and to report to others. They use summative assessments from other teachers to develop learning programmes for new pupils.

The assessments which teachers undertake with individual pupils are central to MARRA. Formative and diagnostic assessment impacts directly upon pupils' learning; it leads towards summative assessment which in turn enables evaluative assessment. Teachers' work with individual pupils is pivotal to school, LEA and national systems and structures such as reaching literacy and numeracy targets and 'raising standards'. One of the most beneficial steps which a teacher can take to enhance assessment and learning is to involve pupils in MARRA.

Analysis

Headington's work on monitoring, assessment, recording, reporting and accountability (MARRA) is used widely in initial teacher training. This extract provides a useful overview of how the Qualified Teacher Status (QTS) standards are linked to the *real* world of assessment, recording and reporting in schools. It is particularly important to chart the virtual concentric circles illustrating the importance of MARRA. In this case, it is interesting to note the priority and status levels operating. You will note we are encouraged to look at assessment from the perspectives of the Secretary of State, LEA, school, parents and finally teachers. While Headington does go on to explore the significance of the learner, it is interesting to compare the approach with that of the Assessment Reform Group (2002). The visual representation of its principles (available at **www.qca.org.uk**) draws the reader's eye immediately to the statement that:

> assessment for learning is the process of seeking and interpreting evidence for use by learners and their teachers to decide where the learners are in their learning, where they need to go and how best to get there.

Practical implications and activities

- Drawing on your experience in school to date, list all the examples of assessment you can think of that are carried out during the school year.
- Try to rank them in order of importance as perceived within the school.
- Try to rank them in order of *usefulness* to the child's learning.
- Do the two lists (points 2 and 3) match? What might be the reasons behind the match or mismatch?

Headington's extract is also helpful in providing insight into the practical uses of the reported outcomes of assessments. While the data will inform local education authority (LEA) and school policy and the resulting targeting of resources, it also interesting to consider the power and influence that this information will hold for parents. Although perhaps not to be encouraged, reports of assessments in the form of National Curriculum levels and test results can be used to form comparisons amongst and between individual children. They also empower parents to ask informed questions about progress being made and help that could be given.

But how accurate is the assessment information that teachers report? Filer and Pollard (2002) issue warnings about the validity of much assessment in schools, since they contest that *the pure objectivity of assessment outcomes is an illusion* (p302). This will be explored further later in the chapter.

What?

This section aims to explore *what* criteria and factors must be considered when exploring how to assess and report on the learning in your classroom.

Before you read the following extract, read:

- **www.qca.org.uk**

Follow the links to Assessment for Learning.

This site provides a wealth of support material and practical ideas around assessment for learning in the primary school.

The preparatory reading above will provide you with a good understanding of the outcomes of the work of the Assessment Reform Group. Its work is underpinned by ten principles that promote an active and participative model for assessment that should:

- be part of effective planning;
- focus on how students learn;
- be central to classroom practice;
- be a key professional skill;
- be sensitive and constructive;
- foster motivation;
- promote understanding of goals and criteria;
- help learners know how to improve;
- develop the capacity for self-assessment;
- recognise all educational achievement.
  (Assessment Reform Group, 2002)

Try to keep the above principles in mind as you read the following short extracts.

Extracts: Black, P, Harrison, C, Lee, C, Marshall, B, Wiliam, D (2002) *Working Inside the Black Box*, **Questioning, p7, Feedback through marking, pp9–10, Peer assessment and self assessment, pp12–14. London: NferNelson**

Questioning
- More effort has to be spent in framing questions that are worth asking, i.e. questions which explore issues that are critical to the development of pupils' understanding.
- Wait time has to be increased to several seconds in order to give pupils time to think and everyone should be expected to have an answer and to contribute to the discussion. Then all answers, right or wrong, can be used to develop understanding. The aim is thoughtful improvement rather than getting it right first time.
- Follow-up activities have to be rich, in that they provide opportunities to ensure that meaningful interventions that extend the pupils' understanding can take place.

Put simply, the only point of asking questions is to raise issues about which the teacher needs information or about which the pupils need to think.
Where such changes have been made, experience has shown that pupils become more active as participants, and come to realise that learning may depend less on their capacity to spot the right answer and more on their readiness to express and discuss their own understanding. The teachers also shift in their role, from presenters of content to leaders of an exploration and development of ideas in which all pupils are involved.

Feedback through marking

Overall, the main ideas for improvement can be summarised as follows:

- Written tasks, alongside oral questioning, should encourage pupils to develop and show understanding of the key features of what they have learnt.
- Comments should identify what has been done well and what still needs improvement, and should give guidance on how to make that improvement.
- Opportunities for pupils to follow up comments should be planned as part of the overall learning process.

The central point here is that, to be effective, feedback should cause thinking to take place.

Implementation of such reforms can change the attitudes of both teachers and pupils to written work: the assessment of pupils' work will be seen less as a competitive and summative judgement and more as a distinctive step in the process of learning.

These developments challenge common expectations. Some have argued that formative and summative assessments are so different in their purpose that they have to be kept apart, and such arguments are strengthened by experience of the harmful influence that narrow 'high-stakes' summative tests can have on teaching. However, it is unrealistic to expect teachers and pupils to practise such separation, so the challenge is to achieve a more positive relationship between the two. This section has set out ways in which this can be done: they can all be used for tests where teachers have control over the setting and the marking, but their application may be more limited for tests where the teacher has little or no control.

- Pupils should be engaged in a reflective review of the work they have done to enable them to plan their revision effectively.
- Pupils should be encouraged to set questions and mark answers to help them, both to understand the assessment process and to focus further efforts for improvement.
- Pupils should be encouraged through peer- and self-assessment to apply criteria to help them understand how their work might be improved.

The main overall message is that summative tests should be, and should be seen to be, a positive part of the learning process. By active involvement in the test process, pupils can see that they can be beneficiaries, rather than victims, of testing because tests can help them improve their learning.

The power behind this small publication lies in its grounding in research, which is given authority through the voices of real teachers engaged in carrying out assessments. The individual learner is at the centre of the purpose of assessment, and is directly involved in the process itself. It is an inescapable reality that all *classroom assessment techniques are social processes that are vulnerable to bias and distortion* (Filer and Pollard, 2002, p302). This being the case, it seems appropriate to immerse assessment in the social reality of the classroom and allow the process to be meaningful for the learner.

Practical implications and activities

- Select a series of lessons or activities that you have taught.
- Revisit them highlighting the assessment strategies you used at the time.
- Can you rework them to include:
  - key critical questions;
  - rich feedback and follow-up activities;
  - opportunities for self and peer assessment?
- What implications are there for the way you plan your lessons?

At this point it might seem that two competing priorities have been identified. Earlier, Headington (2003) gave an insight into the role assessment plays in providing information about performance to a wider audience. Yet Black et al. place all the emphasis on individual learners and their interactions with one another and their teacher. They do acknowledge, however, that *some have argued that formative and summative assessments are so different in their purpose that they have to be kept apart* (Black et al., 2002, p13). I would support them in challenging this notion and propose that, by positively engaging in the summative testing process, children can gain a further appreciation of their performance.

How?

This section explores the *how* of monitoring, recording and reporting. You are challenged to compare in-school monitoring, mainly undertaken through observation, with monitoring at a national level through the use of new data-driven tracking systems .

Personal response

The curriculum which most successfully caters for diversity through differentiation has to accommodate two apparently contradictory requirements – of equity and of individual growth. (Bearne, 1996, p257)

Is this possible? How?

Before you read the following extract, read:

- Clarke, S (2001) *Unlocking Formative Assessment: Practical Strategies for Enhancing Pupils' Learning in the Primary Classroom.* London: Hodder and Stoughton.

This is a seminal, but easy-to-access text that provides a range of insights into the possibilities and challenges of formative assessment.

Personal response

Monitoring strategies – observation

- Recall a time when you were observed in the classroom.
- Was it formal or informal? What factors contributed to it either being formal or informal?
- What happened as a result of the observation?
  Think in terms of your own development as a teacher.
  Think in terms of the children's learning.

The following extract is taken from a PowerPoint presentation.

Extract: Macready, C (2005) *Using Data to Narrow the Achievement Gap*. www.standards.dfes.gov.uk

Using data to raise achievement and narrow the achievement gap
- We all know how important this is
- We all know it can't be done without information:
  - where every child is
  - their recent progress
  - how that progress compares to others'
- Data: a dry word, but critical.
- Our common task : to make school performance data exciting and important for those who need to use it.

What DfES is doing (1)
- Old role : idea, legislation, implementation
- New role : promote innovation, build capacity, help to tackle inequalities, reduce bureaucracy, improve flow of data across the system.
- These principles will be at the heart of our New Relationship with Schools.

What DfES is doing (2)
- England has world-beating data on every pupil and their progress (as I've seen on my travels) and cutting-edge ability to analyse it.
- Publish key information to parents and the public, through School and College Achievement and Attainment Tables and statistical releases.

What DfES is doing (3)
- Through the Pupil Achievement Tracker, offer schools and LEAs more detailed performance data, down to individual pupil level, and target-setting tools.
- Open our data-bases to researchers and other purveyors of school performance information, e.g. Fischer Family Trust.

Doing more : Analysing the Equity Gaps (1)
- DfES statisticians offer us a wide range of analyses to help inform and develop school improvement policies, in general and for particular groups.
- Examples in the next three illustrations:

– improvement by high FSM schools
– attainment by pupils' different ethnic origin
- GCSE etc performance over time by FSM bands.

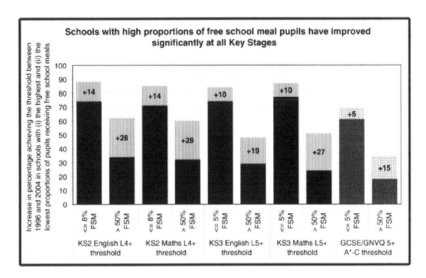

Doing more : analysing the Equity Gaps (2)

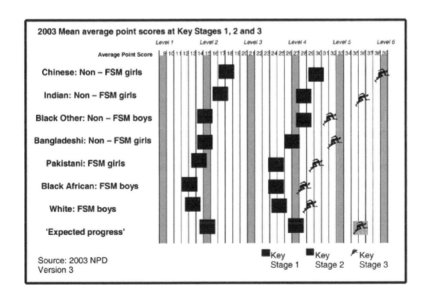

Doing more : analysing the Equity Gaps (3)

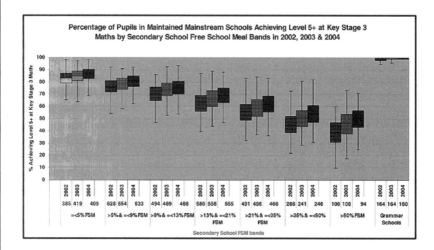

Doing more : analysing the Equity Gaps (4)

Doing more : Contextual Value Added Measures (CVA)

- Aim: to level the playing field between schools in different circumstances
- For all DfES and OfSTED purposes.
- Counting all achievements, through the new inclusive points system QCA devised for secondary school qualifications.
- In PAT 2005, secondary Tables 2006, primary Tables 2007.

The existing Performance Tables Value Added model 'predicts' outcomes based on pupil prior attainment.

A contextualised model predicts outcomes using a range of factors.

But a pupil's value added score remains as the difference between their predicted and their actual result. Pupil VA = Actual Result – Predicted Result

Pupil Characteristics

Pupil Prior Attainment

School Characteristics

Pupil Outcome

How CVA works (1)

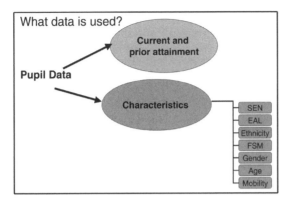

How CVA works (2)

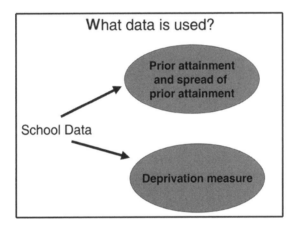

How CVA works (3)

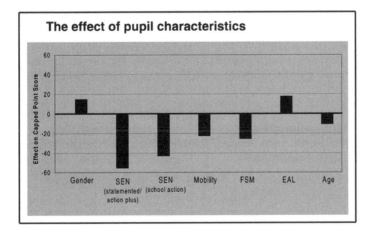

How CVA works (4)

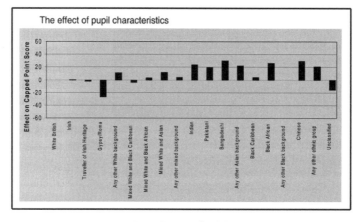

How CVA works (5)

Analysis

The preparatory reading and the above extract could not have provided more contrast in terms of the different interpretations and applications of monitoring and reporting. Macready's current post as Head of School Performance and Accountability is one where she is required to collate and interpret all available monitoring data from schools and LEAs and draw conclusions that can be used to make recommendations for changes in policy in England. Underpinning her role is the belief that data on performance can be used to improve standards in schools. Her presentation clearly acknowledges that this data has not always been used to optimum effect and, thus, the need for the launch of a new *pupil achievement tracker* system. This would be made available to schools and LEAs at the ground level to record individual progress and then to support target-setting. It is interesting to note a clear acknowledgement of the importance of research, by opening DfES databases for analysis by outside audiences.

The huge movement to collect, collate and disseminate data is open to an increasingly wide audience. Website publication of data in all sorts of formats is accessible to experts and interested lay people. However, although education researchers are invited to access and evaluate this information, one questions the use that is made of it. It is perhaps wise to go back to the words of caution of Filer and Pollard (2002, p302).

- Individual pupil performance cannot be separated from the context and social relations from within which they develop.
- Classroom assessment techniques are social processes that are vulnerable to bias and distortion.
- The *results* of assessment take their meaning for individuals via cultural processes of interpretation following mediation by others.

One might argue that Macready's slides above *analysing the equity gaps* are an attempt to acknowledge the context and factors affecting children's performance. True, this might be a starting point, but each learning situation is subject to a wide-ranging set of factors that might include socio-economic, ethnicity and gender differences. Equally, data collated might be influenced by localised factors to do with individual learners, teachers and classrooms.

Filer and Pollard (2002) also point to the fact that the performance data available to us has been interpreted by each person interacting with it – from the teacher in the classroom with personal bias to the statistician providing graphical representations to selected questions. It is useful to reflect for a moment on the number of stages and processes the data has been through, from a single child to that information now represented on *analysing the equity gaps* (slide 4) above.

Nonetheless, this data collection does provide teachers with a wealth of useful information to support their day-to-day work in the classroom. The pupil achievement tracker can be used with individual learners. Macready is suggesting that this is used alongside *contextual value added measures* to help teachers predict the performance of individual children.

While many teachers welcome such supporting predictive and diagnostic tools, these cannot replace the personal and professional interactions, on a minute-by-minute basis in classrooms, that inform immediate action by the teacher to assess and provide targeted support. For all teachers, it is essential that they are able to deploy effective and sensitive observation skills. Stierer, Devereux, Gifford, Laycock and Yerbury (1993) noted:

> the assessment of young children can only be valid and authentic when it is achieved through the gradual building up of a picture of the child based upon evidence collected over a period of time in a range of everyday contexts. (p9)

Practical implications and activities

1. What data can you collect about:
   - a school where you have been on placement?
   - a class that you have taught in that school?
   - a child you have worked with in that particular class?

2. Now that you have access to this information, what changes would you make to the planning and preparation for that class and the child identified?

Ensure that you treat the data and specific details in strictest confidence to preserve the anonymity of the school, class and child concerned.

Summary

This chapter has considered some of the key issues surrounding assessment monitoring, recording and reporting in schools. In considering assessment, you have been challenged to explore the nature and purposes of assessment and how these can be best achieved, depending upon your views about the role of the learner in the learning process. The role of the individual has been further highlighted when considering the ownership and use of performance data, whether this be through teacher observation or through more formal, centrally collated data. But key to all of these areas is the subjective and social context within which we, as teachers, are operating. Education is a social activity and, although this might throw into question the accuracy and interpretation of assessment results, the key to a successful learning experience is grounded in an environment that is rich in human interactions. It is in this context that teachers need to view how they assess, monitor, record and report.

Further reading

Assessment Reform Group (1999) *Assessment for Learning: Beyond the Black Box*. Cambridge: University of Cambridge School of Education.

Conner, C (ed) (1999) *Assessment in Action in the Primary School*. London: Falmer Press.

Hughes, P (2002) *Principles of Primary Education Study Guide*. 2nd edition. London: David Fulton.

Journal of Assessment in Education: Principles, policy and practice.

www.standards.dfes.gov.uk/performance

Section 2: Management, organisation and delivery

4 An introduction to children's learning

By the end of this chapter you should have:

- further considered **why** learning and brain development theories have a powerful contribution to make in the development of your own classroom pedagogy;
- critically evaluated **what** elements of learning theories are evident in current government and contemporary curriculum guidance and practice;
- analysed **how** your own developing principles and values of education are made explicit in your teaching.

Linking your learning

- Jacques, K and Hyland, R (2003) *Achieving QTS. Professional studies: primary phase*, Chapter 5. Exeter: Learning Matters.

Professional Standards for QTS
1.2, 2.4, 3.3.3

Introduction

The parallel chapter, cited above, provides a comprehensive and concise introduction to key theories that relate to children's learning. You are introduced to the behaviourist and cognitivist approaches to learning and teaching, and asked to consider the implications and applications of these in the classroom context. This chapter will take your knowledge and understanding forward by considering how learning is affected by situation and context. A particular emphasis will be placed upon 'affective' domains and influences on learning. Mercer's (2002) article, explored later in the chapter, draws attention to the focus on individual development exemplified in education policy and curriculum developments of the 1980s. More recent curriculum initiatives in primary education, such as *Excellence and Enjoyment* (DfES, 2003b), have begun to promote opportunities that allow for a greater focus on the social and collaborative elements of learning.

New theories relating to learning have won popular appeal in classrooms across the UK. The work of Howard Gardner (1985), with his notion of multiple intelligences, has had huge influence in schools with teachers identifying children who have learning styles that are:

- linguistic;
- logical–mathematical;
- musical;
- bodily–kinaesthetic;
- spatial;

- interpersonal;
- intrapersonal.

Donald Goleman (1996) added to this list by providing an understanding of *emotional intelligence*. The impact of these theories is significant, with teachers planning to teach to preferred learning styles or explicitly to develop these various aspects of their learners.

Personal response

I consider myself to be a .... learner.

Give an example of a successful learning experience you have had that demonstrates this.

As you work through this chapter, it will be useful to reflect on the following two questions.

1. What is the role of the cultural context in the learning?

2. What values and beliefs do I, as a teacher, convey explicitly and implicitly when working with children?

Why?

Before reading the following extract, read:

- Desforges, C (ed) (1995) *An Introduction to Teaching: Psychological Perspectives*. London: Blackwell.

Chapters 1 and 3 provide an analytical overview of the key issues.

Extract: Mercer, N (2002) 'Culture, context and the appropriation of knowledge', in Pollard, A (ed) *Readings for Reflective Teaching*, pp125–27 (Reading 7.9). London: Continuum.

The 1980s was an interesting, if unsettled, period for the study of children's cognition and learning. On the theoretical level, there was a growing unease with theoretical perspectives which focused on individual development to the extent that social and interactional factors in learning and development were marginalized or even ignored. Despite widespread dissatisfaction with the theory and methods of earlier research on the educational attainment of children from different cultural groups (e.g. Jensen, 1967; Bernstein, 1971), more recent research on social experience and children's educational progress (e.g. Tizard and Hughes, 1984; Wells, 1985) made it clear that 'culture' could not be ignored. In particular, it seemed that more attention needed to be paid to the relationship between children's experiences within the cultural environments of home and school, and to the form and content of communication between parents and children and between teachers and children.

But culture and communication were themes that were not clearly or centrally represented within the Piagetian theory which dominated developmental psychology and which had most influence on educational theory and practice [see Reading 7.2]. And so the adequacy of Piagetian theory was questioned (e.g. Walkerdine, 1984; Edwards and Mercer, 1987) and some radical revisions of the Piagetian account of cognitive development were proposed.

Moreover, from the mid-1970s through the 1980s misgivings grew among researchers about how experimental methods had been used to study cognitive development. One important influence was Margaret Donaldson's work (Donaldson, 1978), which showed how strongly experimental results could be influenced by contextual cues carried implicitly within an experimental design or setting. Naturalistic, observational methods thus became rather more popular and experimental methods were devised which were more sensitive to situational factors. It also seemed that Vygotsky's work (e.g. Vygotsky, 1978, [see Reading 7.3]), with its recognition of cultural and linguistic factors on cognitive development and learning might offer a better basis for such observational and experimental research than did Piaget's.

Culture and context thus became necessary and important concepts for the field of cognitive development and learning.

Anthropology, of course, is the discipline with first claims on culture. The eminent anthropologist Geertz (1968, p. 641) offered the following definition 'an historically transmitted pattern of meaning embodied in symbols, a system of inherited conceptions expressed in symbolic form by means of which men [sic] communicate, perpetuate and develop their knowledge about and attitudes towards life'. Geertz's definition seems to me to be compatible with the notion of culture employed by Vygotsky (e.g. 1978, 1981). As Scribner (1985, p. 123) points out 'We find Vygotsky introducing the term 'cultural development' in his discussion of the origins of higher psychological functions and in some contexts using it interchangeably with 'historical development'.' For Vygotsky the concept of culture offers a way of linking the history of a social group the communicative activity of its members and the cognitive development of its children.

The culturally based quality of most learning is represented in the concept of 'appropriation' introduced by Vygotsky's colleague Leont'ev (1981) but taken up and developed by Newman Griffin and Cole (1989). According to Newman *et al.*, it was proposed by Leont'ev as a socio-cultural alternative to Piaget's biological metaphor of 'assimilation' in saying that children appropriate understanding through cultural contact, the point is being made that 'the objects in a child's world have a social history and functions that are not discovered through the child's unaided explorations' (Newman *et al.*, 1989, p. 62). This is more than a complicated way of saying that children do not need to reinvent the wheel. At the simplest level it is arguing that because humans are essentially cultural beings, even children's initial encounters with objects may be cultural experiences and so their initial understandings may be culturally defined. In this sense appropriation is concerned with what children may take from encounters with objects in cultural contexts.

Here is an example from my experience. My daughter Anna, when about nine months old, was offered a toy car to play with by her older brother. Although this was the first time she had seen one at home, she immediately began pushing it along the floor, going 'brrm brrm' as she did so. The explanations for this surprising but conventional response lay in her regular attendance at day nursery. Although not given the opportunity there to handle a car, she had been able to observe an older child playing with one. On being given the car to play with Anna did not need to 'discover' its nature purely through sensori-motor contact to make use of it as a toy. She recognized it as a tool for 'brrm-brrming' because she had appropriated from the older child the culturally based conception and function of the toy. Right from the start, it was a culturally defined object, and not simply a bit of material reality which she had to act on to discover its properties and functions.

The concept of appropriation also incorporates the socio-dynamics of the development of understanding in another, more complex, way, because within the educational process appropriation may be reciprocal. Thus Newman *et al.*, use appropriation to explain the pedagogic function of a particular kind of discourse event where one person takes up another person's remark and offers it back, modified, into the discourse. They show how teachers do this with children's utterances and actions, thereby offering children a recontextualized version of their own activities which implicitly carries with it new cultural meanings. Teachers often paraphrase what children say and present it back to them in a form which is considered by the teacher to be more compatible with the current stream of educational discourse. Teachers also reconstructively recap what has been done by the children in class, so as to represent events in ways which fit their pedagogic framework. By strategically appropriating children's words and actions, teachers may help children relate children's thoughts and actions in particular situations to the parameters of educational knowledge.

The acquisition of knowledge should not be theoretically isolated from the processes by which knowledge is offered, shared, reconstructed and evaluated. As Vygotsky suggested. the concept of culture helps us understand learning as a socio-historical and interpersonal process, not just as a matter of individual change or development. This has particular significance for the study of learning in school, where what counts as knowledge is often quite culturally specific. Culture represents the historical source of important influences on what is learned, how it is learned, and the significance that is attached to any learning that takes place. We likewise need a satisfactory definition of context to deal with learning as a communicative, cumulative, constructive process, one which takes place in situations where past learning is embodied in present learning activity, and in which participants draw selectively on any information which is available to make sense of what they are doing. Only by taking account of these situated qualities of learning can we properly begin to describe how people learn.

Analysis

The article provides an excellent chronological précis of recent theories of learning. It is interesting to relate these developments to the political map of curriculum changes that were being implemented at the same time.

Obviously, the key event was the publication of the National Curriculum (DES, 1989) which was seen as an attempt to raise achievement through the setting of standardised benchmarks. Comparative performance data could be used to form judgements about school effectiveness. The centralised nature of the curriculum content caused controversy and debate, particularly in subject areas that were apparently culturally and socially sensitive. These included English, music, art and, in particular, history. The reader can see the undercurrent of concern about cultural bias, and fear of social manipulation, in the following article extract that claims:

> Baker's [the Secretary of State for Education in 1988] agenda was both racist and nationalistic. History should teach that the British Empire was a great civilising project and that democracy had been born in Britain in the mother of all parliaments. (*Socialist Review*, 1994)

It is true that the above extract takes a particular political stance but, nonetheless, it highlights the apparent contradiction and irony of the period. While the work of Vygotsky (1978) and Leont'ev (1981) highlighted the need for learning to be placed in a social and cultural context for it to be effective and meaningful to the individual, teachers perceived that the opportunity to do this was being denied them.

Further, the extract from Mercer (2002) provides us with another opportunity to acknowledge the importance of the relationship between learner and teacher. This theme, that emerged in Section 1 of this book, is developed here as we consider the notion of reciprocal appropriation. We must expect both learner and teacher to be changed by this engagement in relationship. Current policy developments, such as Workforce Reform (*The Children Act*, DfES, 2004b), will increase the number of adults working with children thus providing the potential for enhanced interactions. This will only be effective, however, if training for adults and teachers in the classroom includes an emphasis upon how to build and sustain relationships with learners.

Practical implications and activities

Taking Mercer's notion of appropriation, as defined in the extract above, find a classroom learning situation to observe. Notice and comment on the exchanges and interactions between learner and teacher where:

- the teacher takes up a child's comment and provides feedback;
- this feedback places the child's comment in another context;
- the exchange is genuinely reciprocal – what is your evidence for this?

What?

Before you read the following extract, read:

- Pollard, A (ed) (2002) 'How we can understand children's development?' *Readings for Reflective Teaching*. London: Continuum.

In this section of his book, Pollard has brought together some of the most influential and current thinkers in the world of child development. This will have provide you with a good all-round introduction to contemporary theories of child development, and their interpretation in the popular classroom applications of people like Claxton (1999) and Gardner (1985). Much of this work is grounded in recent research into brain development and the consequent implications for learning theories.

Extract: *www.routledgefalmer.com/pdf/behaviour.pdf* pp63–65 taken from Mathieson, K and Price, M (2001) *Better Behaviour in Classrooms: A Course of INSET Materials*. London: RoutledgeFalmer.

The triune brain

Human beings are in possession of a three-part (triune) brain. The basic, or reptilian, brain, the emotional brain or limbic system, and the cerebral cortex, or neo-cortex.

The basic or reptilian brain governs our primitive responses and survival instincts. If a threat is perceived, whether real or not, the blood supply retreats from the limbic and neo-cortex systems to fuel the reptilian system.

This prepares us for fight or flight, a flood of hormones, adrenalin being the most recognised, arms our bodies for a physical response. Our heart and breathing rates increase in order to pump up the blood supply to our extremities. Our digestive systems slow down and the sphincters in our bodies close down. We are aware of blood pounding in our ears, butterflies in our stomach, clenching of our teeth, and an involuntary tensing of our major muscles. While this response is aroused, the other parts of the brain are unable to function properly until the stress has subsided or been resolved.

Above the reptilian brain is found the limbic system, or emotional brain, which governs memory, values, and obviously our emotions. This part of the brain provides much of the blueprint that makes each of us unique, a distillation of all our experiences, conditioning and stimuli. This part of the brain validates knowledge as useful to us or not.

At the top of the emotional brain is the reticular activating system (RAS), which acts as a filter from the neo-cortex, validating that which resonates with our emotional 'mind-map', and is personally relevant. In front of this lies the cerebral cortex (neo-cortex) which is divided into right and left hemispheres. The neo-cortex is where we use knowledge and concepts to develop skills. This part of the brain governs language and logic. We use our neo-cortex to work out relationships and patterns of meaning. We create personal models for understanding and developing cognitive skills to solve patterns of meaning.

Communicating with the emotional brain is therefore the vital element in managing behaviour and enabling learning to take place. We must therefore search for ways to make our classrooms as low stress and non-threatening as possible, but also to provide high challenge in order to engage the neo-cortex. Those teachers who provide the 'low-stress-high challenge' classroom will undoubtedly have mastered communication with the emotional brain first and foremost.

Easy to say, but not so easy to achieve. Those pupils whose formative experiences, in the home or at school, have been characterised by difficulty, humiliation and failure are very likely to have a poor self-concept. Their values may be incongruent with those of the school. They may have seen only combative behaviour modelled in the home, and their perennial response to authority, in the first instance, is likely to be hostility or denial, or both. These are the youngsters who present the biggest danger to the emotional well-being of their teachers.

In considering the functions of each part of the brain, it is possible to translate these functions into needs and to provide some insight into how to fulfil these needs.

OHT 2: Effective teachers are skilled at minimising problems

Characteristics of a safe learning environment for all

- minimal threat – high challenge
    routines
    resources
    appropriate tasks
    sharing of purpose

- promotion of a positive self-image
    acknowledge student as an individual
    acknowledge individual strengths
    provide appropriate support for individual needs

- encouragement of high self-esteem
    build in early success/reward
    acknowledge and build on that success
    reminders of previous successes

- engagement of positive emotions
    warm welcome
    showing enthusiasm
    showing approval

OHT 3: Learning needs

The reptilian (basic) brain
- I need to feel safe
    familiar routines
    orderly entrances
    orderly dismissals

> keeping the same seat
> sharing resources safely
>
> - I need to experience success more often than failure
>   start with what I can do
>   celebrate what I can do
>
> - I need to feel noticed
>   say my name
>   welcome me
>
> **Limbic (emotional brain) system**
> - I need to feel respected
>   as a human being
>   as a person of some worth to you
>
> - I need to feel motivated
>   use what I remember
>   understand my values
>   share the purpose of the task
>
> - I need to feel accepted
>   my feelings are important too

Personal response

1. Reflecting on your own personal experiences, can you identify learning events that have engaged your own:

   - reptilian brain;
   - limbic emotional brain;
   - neocortex?

2. Share these with a trusted colleague or friend. What implications does this have for your own learning and teaching styles or strategies?

Analysis

The short extract highlights the importance of acknowledging that learning is multidimensional and, to be effective, needs to draw upon and accommodate all areas of our brain. In contrast with the previous section in this chapter, it is encouraging to see this research impacting on curriculum and school development. For example, current staff development materials to support the implementation of the Primary National Strategy (DfES, 2004a) outline the *principles for learning and teaching* to:

- establish what the learners already know and build on it;
- structure and pace the learning to make it challenging and enjoyable;
- inspire learning through passion for the subject;
- make individuals active partners in their learning;
- develop learning skills and personal qualities.

In giving examples of these principles in practice one can see an attempt to teach to the reptilian brain, with an insistence that teachers should make learners feel *included, valued and secure.* The limbic or emotional element is brought to the fore in the materials in which teachers are asked to build *respectful relationships that take learners' views and experience fully into account.* Third, the neocortex is given prominence in the same materials, which ask teachers to make learning *relevant to learners' wider goals and concerns.* (DfES, 2004a, p15)

One of the key messages to be drawn from the extract is the importance that must be placed upon the learning environment. In creating a space for extension and challenge, an atmosphere where the learner feels secure is paramount.

Practical implications and activities

Hayes (2004) sets out a challenge for teachers, to help them reflect on the learning environment they have created.

> Teachers should put themselves in the child's place. Is the classroom environment stimulating or depressing? How does the attitude of adults (teacher, assistants) serve to motivate or discourage? How do patterns of social interaction, such as friendship patterns, grouping of children and peer support, impinge upon children's appetite to engage with tasks? (Hayes, 2004, p127)

1. Reflect on the most recent classroom you have worked in. Share your answers to Hayes' questions in relation to this context.

2. Identify three practical steps you could take or recommend to facilitate change.

How?

Before you read the extract below, prepare yourself by reading:

- Kyriacou, C (1991) *Essential Teaching Skills,* Chapter 5, 'Classroom climate'. Cheltenham: Stanley Thornes.

Kyriacou provides an extensive and easily accessible list of practical strategies for creating a positive classroom context in which to situate learning. How we go about creating a learning environment that is safe, secure, stimulating and challenging is a matter for individual teachers and the children they are working with. Wragg and Wood (1984) noted that experienced teachers constructed a positive classroom climate in which they personally demonstrated:

- confidence and warmth;
- authority;
- efficiency;
- mobility;
- good use of eye contact;

- a sense of humour;
- clear boundaries and rules.

It is important to realise and accept that, while individual teachers may have preferred ways of working and different personalities, the creation of a positive learning environment will vary each year. Each group of children will be different, school ethos and priorities will shift and, most importantly, it is essential to remember that a group of learners is made up of individuals who are part of the creation process.

Extract: Claxton, G (2002) 'Learning and the development of resilience', in Pollard, A (ed) (2002) *Readings for Reflective Teaching*, pp125–127 (Reading 7.9). London: Continuum.

As the world moves into the age of uncertainty, nations, communities and individuals need all the learning power they can get. Our institutions of business and education, even our styles of parenting, have to change so that the development and the expression of learning power become real possibilities. But this will not happen if they remain founded on a narrow conceptualization of learning: one which focuses on content over process, comprehension over competence, 'ability' over engagement, teaching over self-discovery. Many of the current attempts to create a learning society are hamstrung by a tacit acceptance of this outmoded viewpoint, however watered down or jazzed up it may be. The new science of learning tells us that everyone has the capacity to become a better learner, and that there are conditions under which learning power develops. It is offering us a richer way of thinking about learning, one which includes feeling and imagination, intuition and experience, external tools and the cultural milieu, as well as the effort to understand. If this picture can supplant the deeply entrenched habits of mind that underpin our conventional approaches to learning, the development of learning power, and the creation of a true learning society might become qualities. In this reading, let me summarize the lessons that the new science of the learning mind has taught us.

Learning is impossible without resilience: the ability to tolerate a degree of strangeness. Without the willingness to stay engaged with things that are not currently within our sphere of confident comprehension and control, we tend to revert prematurely into a defensive mode: a way of operating that maintains our security but does not increase our mastery. We have seen that the decision whether, when and how to engage depends on a largely tacit cost-benefit analysis of the situation that is influenced strongly by our subjective evaluations of the risks, rewards and available resources. These evaluations derive from our beliefs and values, our personal theories, which may be accurate or inaccurate. Inaccurate beliefs can lead us to over- or underestimate apparent threats and to misrepresent to ourselves what learning involves.

So when you find people declining an invitation to learn, it is not because they are, in some crude sense, lazy or unmotivated: it is because, for them, at that moment, the odds stack up differently from the way in which their parents or tutors or managers would prefer. Defensiveness seen from the inside, is always rational. If the stick and the carrot don't do the trick, it may be wiser to try to get a clearer sense of what the learner's interior world looks like. Often you will find that somewhere, somehow, the brakes have got jammed. Sensitivity to the learner's own dynamics is always smart.

Some of these beliefs refer to the nature of knowledge and of learning itself. For example, if we have picked up the ideas that knowledge is (or ought to be) clear and unequivocal, or that learning is (or ought to be) quick and smooth, we withdraw from learning when it gets hard and confusing, or when we meet essential ambiguity. Some beliefs refer to hypothetical psychological qualities such as 'ability'. The idea that achievement reflects a fixed personal reservoir of general-purpose 'intelligence' is pernicious, leading people to interpret difficulty as a sign of stupidity, to feel ashamed, and therefore to switch into self-protection by hiding, creating diversions or not trying. Some beliefs determine how much we generally see the world as potentially comprehensible and controllable ('self-efficacy', we called it). High self-efficacy creates persistence and resilience; low breeds a brittle and impatient attitude. Some beliefs forge a connection between self-worth on the one hand and success, clarity and emotional control on the other, making failure, confusion and anxiety or frustration induce a feeling of shame. All these beliefs can affect anyone, but there are a host of others that specifically undermine or disable the learning of certain groups of people, or which apply particularly to certain types of material. For example, girls and boys have been revealed as developing different views of themselves as learners of mathematics.

These beliefs are rarely spelled out, but are transmitted implicitly and insidiously through the kinds of culture that are embodied in the settings that learners inhabit, such as family, school or workplace. Learning messages are carried by a variety of media. The habits and rituals of the culture enable certain kinds of learning and disable others.

The implications of these conclusions for the kinds of learning cultures we create are self-evident. Parents, teachers and managers have to be vigilant, reflective and honest about the values and beliefs which inform the ways they speak, model and organize the settings over which they have control. Inadvertently create the wrong climate and the development and expression of learning power are blocked. Experience in childhood, at home and at school, is particularly important because these early belief systems, whether functional or dysfunctional, can be carried through into people's learning lives as adults.

Analysis

Claxton's article brings us back to the discussion of the later part of Chapter 1. In revisiting the recent history of priorities in education, Claxton reinforces the view that subject content and teacher delivery have been the focus of work in schools. His work resonates with that of Hayes (2004), who supports putting the emphasis back onto the processes of learning and teaching.

The ability to succeed in developing ways of learning depends on a range of factors. Claxton highlights the need for teachers to reflect on the model that they are providing and the values and beliefs they are promoting, perhaps implicitly. While Claxton appears to be focusing on the teachers' beliefs and values around learning, he only hints at their beliefs around personal worldviews. Arthur, Davison and Lewis (2005, p31) suggest that when it comes to teachers' values:

> what counts most in their professional practice is the extent to which they can successfully apply them in their work so that positive attitudes and dispositions inform and influence the way pupils work and learn.

Arthur *et al.* advocate that teachers should promote a set of values to which they wish their learners to subscribe. Although their discussion goes on to elaborate upon a set of values, and insists that pupils are part of the process of identification of these shared values, this quotation does hint at the immense power and influence at the teacher's disposal. Claxton is keen to reinforce this message by urging teachers to make explicit their values, but he goes further. He insists that teachers be *vigilant* about how their beliefs and values are imbued in their teaching, and how this might promote or constrain the learner.

The sense of trust that will evolve from a teacher–child relationship in which values and expectations are explicit will allow the learner to feel safe and confident. This echoes research into the brain and learning, mentioned above, that has highlighted the need of the learner to feel safe, respected and consulted. It is in this climate that a learner can develop the resilience that Claxton emphasises as being crucial to success. Learning is about meeting the new and unfamiliar, taking risks and making mistakes, so that children can make sense of the content of their learning so that it is relevant and owned. This takes motivation and determination, and the resilience to try the new, and keep on trying.

Personal response

1. Think of yourself as the learner and try to recall learning experiences where you were:

   - afraid to try and perhaps did not even attempt the task or gave up quickly;
   - anxious at the task set but worked to master this new knowledge or skill.

2. Can you identify what role your teacher played during both experiences? What was your relationship like with your teacher during both experiences?

Summary

This chapter has explored some of the contemporary theories of learning and their popular applications to classroom pedagogy. Once again, the theme of teacher–child relationship is highlighted as being at the core of all successful learning experiences. The works of Bruner (1986) and Vygotsky (1978) place great emphasis on the role of the more knowledgeable *other* in providing the scaffolding on which to build new experiences. Gardner (1985) and Goleman (1996) point to the need for teachers to tap into the varying styles and domains in which learners operate. Above all, the message is that teachers and children need to co-construct the learning, in an environment that is safe and experimental. Teachers need to take a principled stance, however, and ensure that they are open and explicit about what they hold to be important. They need to enter the learning relationship with their set of values and expectations known to all, but also to be prepared genuinely to engage in change and development. The relationship between learner and teacher must be reciprocal in an active and purposeful sense. This will open the way for the development of resilience in the learners, and in this world of challenge and change, perhaps in the teacher too.

Further reading

Blandford, S (2005) *Remodelling Schools*. London: Pearson.

Bruner, J (1986) *Actual Minds – Possible Worlds*. Cambridge MA: Harvard Educational Press.

Claxton, G (ed) (1997) *Hare Brain, Tortoise Mind. Why Intelligence Increases When You Think Less*. London: Fourth Estate.

Vygotsky, L.S (1978) *Mind in Society: The Development of Higher Psychological Processes*. Cambridge, MA: Harvard University Press.

5 Managing the classroom for learning

By the end of this chapter you should have:

- further considered **why** classroom management and effective learning are inextricably linked;
- critically evaluated **what** constitutes classroom management, including an emphasis on managing the other adults in your classroom;
- analysed **how** your own developing pedagogy and educational values provide a foundation from which you can consider how to manage the learning in your classroom.

Linking your learning

- Jacques, K and Hyland, R (2003) *Achieving QTS. Professional studies: primary phase*, Chapter 6. Exeter: Learning Matters.

Professional Standards for QTS
3.3.1, 3.3.3, 3.3.7, 3.3.8

Introduction

Waterson's chapter in Jacques and Hyland (2003) is successful in drawing attention to the practical manifestations of different philosophies of learning, and to how these are visible in the ways teachers organise and manage the learning in their classrooms. This chapter will take your knowledge and understanding forward, by considering how contemporary development theories discussed in the previous chapter need to be influential, in the light of current government policy and legislation. A particular emphasis will be placed on Workforce Reform developments (WAMG, 2003) and the OFSTED (2003a, 2003b) inspection framework for primary schools.

The previous chapter highlighted the importance of children feeling safe and secure in order for effective learning to take place. Within such an environment they can successfully be supported in taking risks and developing resilience. The classroom management and organisation implications of these basic requirements are explored further.

For learning to be effective, children need to be able to construct and own the knowledge they are creating. This necessitates a classroom that is active and participative so that learning can be celebrated as *understanding things differently – not just remembering more information* (Jessel, 2000, p4). The management style and resulting methods of organisation you adopt need to allow the children to construct their own meanings and, in so doing, to have space for active engagement and risk-taking.

As you work through this chapter, it will be useful to reflect on the following two questions.

1. What opportunities do new government initiatives open up for more constructive approaches in the classroom?

2. How far can the management style employed in the classroom support the development of resilience?

Why?

Before you read the following extract, read:

- Hughes, P (2000) *Principles of primary education study guide* (2nd edition), 'Classroom organisation and management: the effective teacher'. London: David Fulton.

This chapter provides a practical overview of the key considerations.

Extract: Laslett, R and Smith, C (2002) 'Four rules of class management', in Pollard, A (ed) (2002) *Readings for Reflective Teaching*, pp218–21 (Reading 11.4). London: Continuum.

The skills of successful classroom management can be reduced to 'four rules', attention to which should enable all teachers to improve efficiency and harmony in their classrooms.

Rule one: get them in
The first rule requires attention to planning the start of each lesson. The process of beginning a lesson smoothly and promptly involves greeting, seating and starting.

Greeting Simply by being present before the class arrives, the teacher establishes his role as host, receiving the class on his territory and, by implication, on his terms (Marland, 1975). Apart from the vital practical advantage of being able to check that the room is tidy, materials are available, displays are arranged and necessary instructions or examples are written on the blackboard, being there first allows the teacher to underline quietly his authority by deciding when the class comes into the room.

Seating Just how seating is arranged must depend on the type of lesson to be taught, and the type of classroom furniture. Whether using traditional serried ranks of desks or less formal group tables, each teacher needs to establish who sits where.

Starting Every lesson should start with some activity that keeps each child quietly occupied in his own place. What type of activity depends very much on the age and ability of the child and the nature of the lesson. Ideally, the work should involve reinforcement of previously acquired skills, particularly those required for the lesson which is about to be taught. Establishing a routine will require setting specific tasks and providing detailed verbal and written instruction. Having settled the class to work in this way, the temptation to leave them at it must be avoided.

Rule two: get them out
However, before considering the content of the lesson, the second rule which needs to be mastered is how to conclude the lesson and dismiss the class. If this seems a strange

order of priorities, it is worth remembering that if most disciplinary problems arise from a poor start to the lesson, hard-won control is most frequently lost and learning wasted at the end of lessons.

Concluding Learning that has taken place during a lesson can often be wasted if an opportunity is not taken to reinforce what has been taught by a summary and brief question session. It is no use trying to do that over the heads of children who are still working or who are busy collecting exercise books. So at three minutes before the presumed end of the lesson, 'as precisely as that' (Marland, 1975), or at whatever time is judged necessary, work should stop, leaving an opportunity for the collection of materials, putting books away and some revision and recapitulation of the lesson.

Dismissing Once the bell does go, there is need for an established, orderly routine which ensures that the class gets beyond the door without the teacher having to spend time clearing debris from the floor or readjusting the lines of desks. If this can be done without recourse to sending out one section or row at a time, such informality is welcome. Traditional verbal prompting, 'arms folded, sitting up straight', may still have its place, however.

It is also important to remember that classes are never just leaving one place, they are going on to another. Children need to be cued in to their next activity.

Rule three: get on with it

'It' refers to the lesson itself – its content, manner and organization. Momentum is the key to determining the content of a lesson, its variety and pace.

Content Variety is needed within a lesson to maintain interest, curiosity and motivation. Activities planned for the start and finish, as suggested above, will go some way towards achieving these aims. However, there is also a need to plan for some variety within the main body of the lesson. Alternating preferred activities with more boring ones, mixing familiar work with new learning, and balancing quiet individual work with more active group tasks can all help keep a lesson moving (Sloane, 1976). It is essential, however, that variety should not become confusion. Each activity should be clearly specified and the teacher's expectations clarified so that each child knows what he should be doing and when he should be doing it.

Pace is also helped by breaking up a topic into several smaller units of learning. It can also help to have as a target the intention that every child should have something finished, something marked in every lesson. Though often unattainable, such an aim does direct attention to the importance of immediate feedback and reinforcement in helping children to learn (Stott, 1978).

The momentum or flow of classroom industry is of great importance to discipline, as interruptions lead to loss of energy and interest on the part of pupils and teachers (Tanner, 1978; Rutter *et al.*, 1979).

Manner Classroom atmosphere is a term frequently used, but rarely analysed. Here again, however, what might at first be thought to result from 'personality' can be described as a series of skills. Similarly, positive interaction between teacher and class can be traced to the way in which they communicate with each other. The skills involved in creating a good classroom atmosphere are really a series of mechanisms to regulate what goes on in the classroom.

Behaviour does seem to be better and atmosphere brighter where ample praise is used in teaching (Hopkins and Conrad, 1976). Praise needs to be natural and sincere and should never become dull and routing. It is a good idea to try to think of at least six synonyms for 'good' and to use them appropriately. 'Great', 'superb', 'fine', 'splendid', 'remarkable' are some examples, or use more colloquial expressions such as 'ace', 'knockout' or 'cracker', if they come naturally. Similarly, 'nice' is a word so often used, when children would surely be more stimulated to know that their work was 'delightful', 'imaginative', 'beautiful', 'interesting', 'original' or 'fascinating'.

The way the teacher talks to the class reflects his attitude to them not only in what is said, but how it is said. Facial expression and tone of voice are as important to communication as making sure that attention is gained, by getting the class to stop work and listen carefully to what has to be said. It follows that what has to be said should be clear, simple and important enough to merit stopping the lesson.

The old adage, 'quiet teacher, quiet class' contains good advice, but should be followed with some reservation; 'inaudible teacher, insufferable class' may also be true. Adequate volume is an essential to being understood and it may help if teachers assume that in any class there is very likely to be at least one child with some hearing loss.

Emphasizing the importance of using your eyes to communicate, is recommended by Marland (1975). Two or three sentences on a theme should be addressed to one child in one part of the room. As another idea is developed, the teacher shifts his gaze to another child in another part of the room, then focuses on a third for the next theme. This approach should help develop a 'feel' for what is going on in the different areas of the classroom. This is how to develop the traditional teacher's eyes in the back of the head.

Organization In any given subject, every class is a mixed-ability group. Whether dealing with high flyers or low achievers, teachers must allow for the fact that some children will work more rapidly and accurately than others. On the way to the ideal of individualizing educational programmes for all their pupils, teachers can start by splitting their class into groups. The amount and difficulty of work demanded from each group can then be related to their abilities in that particular subject. There are three ways of doing this – by rota, quota or branching.

Rota, as in rotation of crops, refers to groups moving round the classroom from one activity to another. The development of learning centres is essential to this approach. These are areas of the classroom using alcoves, bookshelves or simply tables arranged to provide an environment for the accomplishment of a particular instructional purpose (Lemlech, 1979). They can be used for the practice of particular skills, gathering further information, extending experience or for instructional recreation.

Quota, similarly requires the teacher to work out an appropriate amount of work to be completed during a session by each group. Each child has an assignment card or booklets, which becomes a record of work completed as it is checked by the teacher. This system can be simply an extension of the rota system with individual requirements, such as reading to the teacher, handwriting or spelling practice being added.

Branching, involves starting all the class together on a particular activity, doing an exercise from the board or working together from a textbook, then, as this is completed, 'branching' groups into different activities or areas of the room. For the quicker workers, who are likely to finish the common activity first, there may need to be a number of further pieces of work.

Rule four: get on with them

The temptation to misbehave is lessened where teachers and children get on well together. Many of the points already mentioned will help build a good pupil-teacher relationship, based on skilful, confident teaching geared to children's specific needs (Wallace and Kauffman, 1978). To further develop mutual trust and respect, the teacher also needs to show an awareness of each child as an individual and a sensitivity to the mood of the class as a whole. The teacher needs to know who's who and what's going on.

Who's who? Once a child's name is known, discipline is immediately easier because requests or rebukes can be made more personal. Recognition also implies interest on the part of the teacher. It is easy to learn the names of the best and worst children, but less easy to remember those who do not attract attention to themselves. The attention is needed just as much, and sometimes more.

A daily chat, however brief, about something not connected with lessons can be a source of insight as well as a way of establishing rapport. It might be said that a chat a day, keeps trouble at bay! As with praise, personal interest must be natural and genuine, not merely assumed.

What's going on? Few classes of children are likely to be so purposefully malevolent as to set out on a planned campaign of disruption. Group misbehaviour is more likely to build up from a series of minor incidents. It is necessary therefore for teachers to acquire a sensitivity to group responses. 'The key to developing this talent lies in a combination of monitoring, marking and mobility' (Brophy and Evertson, 1976).

Frequently scanning the class, even while helping one individual should enable the teacher to spot the first signs of trouble quickly and intervene firmly but quietly. Often, merely moving to the area from which louder voices are indicating some distraction can refocus abstention on the work in hand. The mild personal rebuke addressed to an individual can be far more productive than a formal public warning.

Marking work in progress is not only a good way of giving immediate feedback, it is also a natural form of contact. Rather than reprimanding the child who is not concentrating on this work, offering help and advice may be the best way to return his attention to the task in hand.

Mobility is needed to avoid teachers becoming desk-bound by queues waiting for attention, which can screen inactivity elsewhere in the classroom and themselves become social gatherings and a potential source of noise and distraction. It is essential to develop a routine, which enables children to find help from each other if the teacher is occupied, or which provides them with alternative purposeful activities while waiting for advice or correction. This will free the teacher to move around the room, sharing his time and interest, adding all the time to his awareness of personalities and problems.

It is this combination of activities that enables the responsive teacher to judge correctly the times for serious endeavour or light-hearted amusement.

Analysis

The article provides a clear and direct set of guidelines for beginning teachers, to help them focus on the key essentials of classroom management. The guidelines are based upon the view that order, clarity, pace and efficiency will allow the teacher to establish a relationship with the children. Statements concerning teachers' authority over their territory might lead one to assume that there is a traditional agenda operating in classrooms such as those advocated in this extract. It is perhaps difficult to hear the learner's voice in such classrooms.

Although Laslett and Smith appear in many ways to be advocating a teacher-led model they do place considerable emphasis upon the importance of a positive relationship between teacher and learner. Their practical strategies are worth noting, particularly the call for personal interest to be genuine. Kyriacou (1991, p10) takes this further by noting the importance of 'mutual respect and rapport'.

An overarching theme in this extract is the active nature of effective teaching and classroom management. Laslett and Smith (2002) point to a profession that demands that its members be physically (and emotionally) fit and not desk-bound. The classroom needs to be planned with the movement of all in mind. If learning is to be active, children need to be encouraged to problem-solve and, in so doing, to move around the room gathering resources and collaborating with fellow learners. The teacher is part of this activity and needs to be able to move to where learning is happening, to support, scaffold and assess the learning taking place. Hughes's work (2000) provides a useful insight for student teachers into factors they need to consider when establishing the classroom: active learning is encouraged, but it brings with it potential health and safety issues.

Practical implications and activities

Hughes's (2002) list of safety considerations includes:

- avoid congestion in high traffic areas;
- make sure instructional support can be seen by everyone;
- make sure children are always visible;
- create individual space for children to store their personal belongings.

These have been selected because of their importance in supporting the management of an active learning environment.

Draw a plan of your last placement classroom, and reflect on the above points.

1. What recommendations for changes would you suggest in order to encourage active learning?
2. Was there room for a teacher's desk? If so, how was it used?
3. What does this tell you about the style of learning promoted in this classroom?

While this section focuses on the physical presentation of the classroom and associated safety considerations, it is also worth recalling the previous chapter. Children learn more effectively if they feel safe and secure and, although this must include physical safety, it is also about the extent to which they feel able to take conceptual risks through hypothesising and problem solving.

What?

Before you read the following extract, read:

- Worton, C (2005) 'Classroom approaches and organisation', in English, E and Newton, L *Professional studies in the primary classroom.* London David Fulton.

Extract: McNamara, S and Moreton, G (1997) *Understanding Differentiation*, pp77–79. London: David Fulton.

Differentiation by classroom organisation
In our model, 'differentiation by classroom organisation' means a set of structures that are designed to organise the children into working with each other and supporting each other. We have specified the structures which we have found to offer a clear focus on helping children to work together.

Most primary teachers use groupwork in their classrooms. Few primary teachers use the structures outlined in this chapter. As many researchers have found (Galton, 1980, and Bennet, 1976), if children are simply told to make groups of four, given a collaborative task and then left to get on with it, they will either be unable to do the task because they fall out with each other or they will get the task done and some members of the group will have contributed very little. The reason why some members contribute very little is that showing what you know in front of a group can be very risky. You risk failing and being made fun of.

The framework below outlines the different types of risk that face children in the classroom. Different tasks create different levels of risk.

1. High ambiguity – low risk; example, complex maths problem in apprenticeship situation.
2. Low ambiguity – high risk; example, small construction toy, only one way to put it together carried out in a group which itself is being watched.
3. High ambiguity – high risk; example, discussion on controversial issue in large group, teacher present.

4. Low ambiguity – low risk; example, simple maths addition, conforms to rules, carried out routinely.

There are some learning situations where the risk is to do with speaking out in front of other people although the task is fairly straightforward e.g. 'yes' or 'no' answers. There are other situations where the task is risky because there is no right answer, e.g. discussion or research. Unless teachers are aware of this they can set a task where both the content and the performing of the task carry a high risk, e.g. role play of an historical situation which requires children to act in front of others whilst dealing with newly acquired factual knowledge. The children have to acquire the confidence and skill to deal with such high risk situations but they need to do so step by step through skills training and confidence building structures.

The structures we recommend in this chapter offer low risk to children in the learning situation whilst enabling the teacher to deliver the same curriculum strand to all the children at the same time. This enables the teacher to have a clear map of the content covered by a whole class while at the same time giving access to the content to all of the children. Through their observations of children the authors recognise that speaking out in front of the whole class is the most risky thing for learners to do when the result could be humiliation. However, participation in a whole class learning experience is one of the most affirming and motivating experiences as it results in personal recognition and affiliation to the class group. This leads to cohesion and a class that is a pleasure to teach.

The structures offer the children the opportunity to practise being in the large group but with very low ambiguity and therefore gain experience and expertise in whole group participation. This will help them to cope with whole group, higher ambiguity situations. Alongside this whole group experience, small group work can give the necessary practice, skill development and confidence for children both to deal with the scary feelings of talking out in front of the whole class and to gain the support and benefits that small groups can provide. The benefits are the same as in pair work, i.e. independence as a learner, support through talk and valuing your achievements, but these benefits can be multiplied in small group work. It is our belief that the pair is the safest place and therefore small group work needs to be built up from pairs. This is done in several ways.

Pair work can go some way towards building confidence and reducing risk but it doesn't give any practice in performing in the larger arena. For some children being in a class of thirty is in fact a very high risk activity. The carousel provides the opportunity for the children to work with the whole class in a highly structured and safe manner as they are always in a pair. The children work with many others in the class but only have to work with one partner at any one time The change of partners is highly structured and offers no risk to their self-esteem.

All children need to have the risk reduced when they are dealing with new knowledge or concepts that challenge their old knowledge. The structure of jigsawing was developed by Eliot Aronson (1978) to reduce the risk involved in research. In this structure children are able to find out information about small parts of a larger subject thus sharing the responsibility whilst finding out new knowledge. The structure still allows all the children to learn and share in the whole subject whilst only being responsible for a smaller part.

Another structure used is snowballing. This is when pairs join into fours and then into eights. This means that the risk involved in children sharing their current ideas and concepts is reduced. The result is that the risk of not getting a correct response is shared among the group. Figure 6.1 summarises three group structures: carousel, jigsaw and snowball.

- **Snowball** safe because it starts with pairs, information is 'collected' as pairs form a four
- **Jigsaw** reduce risk, share knowledge and find out knowledge from 'experts'
- **Carousel** explain and re-tell current understanding, conceptual understanding developed

Figure 6.1 Group structures for learning

Through these approaches we believe that children can gain access to the curriculum in a way that does not make them feel de-motivated as it gives all children an experience of success as learners and preserves their feelings of self-worth. By working this way we have found that it then becomes possible to use traditional differentiation methods such as ability groupings on some occasions without children suffering the labelling, drop in self-esteem and de-motivation which are common results of long term setting of children.

Analysis

When considering classroom management, one of the key decisions to be made concerns how to organise the children for the learning. Is the focus going to be on whole-class, group or individual work? Is there going to be a mixture of arrangements, and if so, what are the criteria by which the children are to be grouped? Pollard (2005), drawing on a range of research, has highlighted a number of ways of grouping, by:

- task groups;
- teaching groups;
- seating groups;
- collaborative groups;
- age groups;
- attainment groups;
- interest groups;
- friendship groups.

McNamara and Moreton (1997) explore the notion of progressive versus traditional teaching organisation. They suggest that mixed ability grouping is indicative of progressive teaching styles, whereas grouping or streaming by ability suggests a more traditional philosophy.

Whichever method of grouping is employed, McNamara and Moreton suggest that teachers give considerable attention to the *risk* element for the children who are participating. As they indicate above, there are a number of types of risk that may be faced by children working in a group situation.

Practical implications and activities

From your own experience of observing or teaching, can you recall activities that were:

- high ambiguity – low risk?
- low ambiguity – high risk?
- high ambiguity – high risk?
- low ambiguity – low risk?

1. Which children were able to succeed in the different contexts?
2. How could you have changed the activity or the grouping to allow more children to participate?

Current government initiatives to reform the education workforce (DfES, 2004b) will necessarily involve more adults working with classes and groups of children in the classroom. This will provide teachers with new opportunities to review the organisational strategies that they employ. On the one hand, one might argue that the increased number of adults will mean a greater number of high risk activities are possible without compromising children's perception of security. However, it will be essential that shared values, understandings and messages are consistently conveyed by all adults to prevent children from experiencing anxiety and confusion. Consequently, it will be important that teachers work, and share ownership of the planning of the learning, with support staff.

How?

Before you read the following extract, read:

- WAMG (2003) *Guidance for Schools on Cover Supervision.*
  Available at **www.teachernet.gov.uk**

This short article provides an overview of how schools might implement the Workforce Reform policy to allow teachers guaranteed non-contact time during the school day.

Extract: Hayes, D (2004) 3rd edition, *Foundations of Primary Teaching*, pp191–93. London: David Fulton.

Managing learning

Forms of management

It is imprudent to think that because the classroom organisation has been carried out efficiently in advance of the lesson, everything will proceed without a hitch. The best teachers not only organise but ensure that they manage classroom affairs (monitoring,

---

intervening, guiding, assessing) so as to ensure the most favourable conditions for learning. The concept of effective management is now strongly rooted in classroom practice and poor management is likely to result in weaker teaching and underachievement.

Management is derived from the root 'manage', a word we use in a variety of expressions that emphasise a successful outcome. Examples of how the word is used include:

- 'I managed to get there on time.' That is, I succeeded in meeting the deadline.
- 'She managed the final question.' That is, that she had sufficient knowledge to ensure success.
- 'He managed to control the class.' That is, he had the ability to cope successfully.

The use of such expressions points to three different aspects of management that teachers need to take into account: (a) time management; (b) information management; (c) human management. For example, in the expressions noted above, there are underlying assumptions about each of the three forms of management:

- That the person has taken responsibility to meet the deadline (time management)
- That the person needed to be sufficiently well informed to meet a requirement (information management)
- That the person coped with the challenges presented by a class of children (human management).

The significance of these three elements for teachers, who need to meet deadlines (such as finishing lessons on time), be well informed (in particular, to have good subject knowledge) and cope with pupils (establishing and maintaining order) is considerable. A summary of the practical implications helps to underline these points.

- *Time management.* Good time management establishes a framework for working, both within individual lessons and across a whole day. It allows for the quirks of classroom life, accommodates the unexpected and ensures that time is used appropriately. This does not mean that every moment is accounted for in the planning process or that pupils have to keep their 'noses to the grindstone' but rather that time is utilised purposefully and effectively. More information about time management can be found below.
- *Information management.* Good information management ensures that the teacher has a high level of subject knowledge and knows how to access additional sources as required. Teachers who are good at managing information will have the confidence to share ideas with pupils, show interest in their discoveries, monitor their understanding and encourage them to find out more.
- *Human management.* This involves finding ways of relating effectively to pupils and assistants, and engaging them in the teaching and learning process. Human management is facilitated by clarifying boundaries of behaviour for pupils, using stimulating teaching approaches and presenting ideas in a comprehensible form. Good human managers respect pupils' genuine concerns and make allowances for their failings. The learning environment is characterised by a sense of wellbeing, mutual respect, high expectation and undisguised celebration of progress.

Organisation and management are mutually dependent for successful teaching and learning. A good organiser and poor manager promises much and delivers little. A poor organiser and good manager make the most of the situation despite the low level preparation. A good organiser and a good manager not only promise much in advance but make the fullest use of teaching opportunities for the benefit of every pupil.

Analysis

Hayes' discussions stress that managing a class is a multidimensional process that extends beyond a popular conception of classroom management that focuses on behaviour and resources.

Personal response and reflection

Using Hayes's subheadings below, rate yourself out of ten for management in your own personal life:

- time management;
- information management;
- human management.

Are these gradings reflected in your work in the classroom?

It is interesting to explore the links between your own personal management and how this transfers into your work in schools. Hayes notes that a teacher who is managing effectively will be confident and interested, showing concern for well-being and a genuine respect for the children they are teaching. The *Framework for Inspecting Schools* (OFSTED, 2003b) encourages the inspectors to assess the extent to which teachers:

- plan effectively;
- interest, encourage and engage pupils;
- use methods and resources that enable pupils to learn effectively;
- make effective use of time;
- promote equality of opportunity.

While it is easy to see the link between these selected criteria and classroom management, there is no mention of the need to develop an ethos where children feel positively valued and the teacher is demonstrating respect and genuine interest in the children as learners. Perhaps the greatest mismatch is that OFSTED does not seem to acknowledge the importance of a safe, but risk-taking environment, where children can develop resilience as learners. The emphasis, as presented in the inspection framework, is on output from the learners, and lacks a focus on processes of learning.

A key area of resonance in all classroom management texts and OFSTED documentation is the importance of managing the additional adults who may be working alongside the teacher. Historically, additional adults in the room may have been viewed as the teacher's 'spare pair of hands', unless they had specific expertise in supporting individual children with identified needs. It is becoming more and more usual to see other expert adults working alongside the teacher, and this increases in areas such as primary modern foreign languages, music and physical education. Kendall (2000) stresses the importance for student teachers of being clear about the various roles and responsibilities of those additional adults they will be working with in schools. As the workforce in schools expands, this must remain a priority for staff development.

The *Guidance for Schools on Cover Supervision*, issued by the Workforce Agreement Monitoring Group (WAMG, 2003) and supported by the DfES and most relevant trade unions, is designed to give some support to schools as they move towards the workforce reform that will provide guaranteed release time for primary school teachers. The guidance makes it clear that *cover supervision occurs when there is no active teaching taking place* (WAMG, 2003, note 2). It seems contradictory to suggest that this can lead to effective learning, since it is important that learning is active, with an informed and immediate response to performance that can be used to inform future learning.

Summary

This chapter has focused on issues that will be important as the primary school workforce changes to respond to the Workforce Reform agenda (DfES, 2003a) and the necessary remodelling that will be the consequence. Alongside this, the recently re-elected Labour government is pushing ahead with its policy for extended schools. This is largely an immediate response to *Every Child Matters* (DfES, 2003c) which makes provision for increased social and educational facilities for children. Part of this key legislation is to provide for an extended 8a.m.–6p.m. school day to offer greater levels of quality childcare provision. If successful, children will benefit from the five outcomes that are to:

- be healthy;
- stay safe;
- enjoy and achieve;
- make a positive contribution;
- achieve economic well-being.

One of the most immediate and visible impacts upon children will be that they will be working with a much greater range and number of adults on a day-to-day basis. A key theme of this chapter has been to stress the importance of shared values, understandings and methodologies for all adults working with a group of children. If *Every Child Matters* is to succeed and help all children achieve, stay safe and enjoy, it is vital that they can be active in their learning, take risks and develop ownership and resilience. The message for new and training teachers is that you must include all adults in the learning organisation and management of your classroom.

Further reading

Blandford, S (2005) *Remodelling schools*. London: Pearson.

English, E and Newton, L (2005) *Professional studies in the primary school*. London: David Fulton.

Herne, S, Jessel, J and Griffiths, J (2000) *Study to teach*. London: Routledge.

importance of the affective in learning (see Chapter 4), give teachers the legitimate justification to raise the profile of the relationships that exist in their classrooms.

Personal response

1. Reflect on the attributes of someone who has taught you whom you would term *a good teacher*. Brainstorm the characteristics you can recall. Highlight those words that describe your relationship.
2. Is there an obvious link between quality of teaching and learning, and the relationship with the teacher?

What?

Before you read the following extract, read:

- OFSTED (2003a) *Handbook for inspecting primary nursery and schools.* Available at **www.OFSTED.gov.uk**

This booklet provides guidance for those carrying out inspections.

Extract: HMI (1994) 'Characteristics of good practice', in Pollard, A and Bourne, J. (ed) *Teaching and learning in the primary school*, pp120–22. London: Routledge.

Characteristics of the work in the classroom
The examples of good practice differ in their curricular content but there are some features common to the way the children were working.

- In almost all cases first impressions were of an informality which typifies many primary classrooms. Closer investigation showed that the freedoms were not there merely by chance. They had been adopted for a variety of interrelated reasons; for example, on those occasions when children were permitted to move about the classroom so that they had access to the materials they needed and in order that they could use reference books, they were being taught, at the same time, to select from a range of materials, to behave responsibly, and to persevere with the task in hand while showing a proper consideration for others working in the same room. By these and other means a sense of self discipline was being nurtured.
- The children were keenly interested in the work. Their commitment to what they were doing extended beyond the more obviously enjoyable aspects of the practical activities. It was sustained in their efforts to achieve a high standard of 'end product', whether that was to be in the form of written recording, one or other of the modes of pictorial representation, a dramatic presentation, or a combination of these things.
- According to their age and ability and in various aspects of good practice the children were being taught to listen carefully and to speak clearly and articulately. In many cases the discussions arising from the work centred on the similarities and differences of things they had observed, the patterns they had noticed and, again according to the children's ability, the validity of the generalisations which could be drawn from

their experiences. They were encouraged to read for pleasure and for information. Their written work caused them to use a variety of styles to meet a range of purposes and, in this matter, fluency and legibility were given fitting attention.

The high quality of teaching was the strongest feature common to all the examples in this publication. As might be expected there were variations in the teaching styles reflecting the needs of the situation and the personality of individual teachers. Nevertheless there were common characteristics in the intentions and the methods used.

It was evident that the teachers had a sound knowledge of their pupils' social and cultural backgrounds and this enabled them to draw upon each child's experience in order to lead them on to further learning and, in some cases, to choose starting points for studies likely to interest the majority of children.

A dominant factor in the achievement of high standards was the strength of commitment on the part of the teachers to ensure that pupils were making progress. It was characteristic that the teachers consistently faced the question, 'Is that a sufficiently high standard for that particular child?' Their answers – and perhaps even their readiness to ask the question – revealed a firm grasp of the long-term aims and the more immediate objectives of the curriculum. The various teaching methods used were all geared to making the work suitably challenging so that individually the children consolidated what they were learning and reached forward to tackle the next stage. Whether teaching the class as one unit, organising groups, or channelling special work to individuals, the matter of progression was kept in mind. Methods of evaluation and records of attainment were used as an aid to planning future activities. Challenges were set so that the work was neither too easy nor too difficult for the children. In itself, this well-matched work was a notable achievement but it was heightened by the fact that a sense of self-assessment had spread to the children. The 'climate of assessment' was accepted and many of the pupils were able to speak lucidly about what they had learned, give reasons why they were engaged in certain activities, explain what they planned to do next and, in many cases, express a reasoned view of how well they were doing. Furthermore, the teachers weighed the children's responses carefully according to individual differences in ability so that praise was not given lightly or attributed to slipshod or mediocre work. Children were nevertheless commended when their work and efforts deserved it.

In all the examples of good practice the educational objectives were firmly established. Some had been made explicit in the school's guidelines or the teacher's schemes of work; some, such as those relating to orderliness and effort, were implicit in the ethos of the school and were given expression in the teaching styles. This clear view of objectives had not in any way reduced the flexibility of the teaching arrangements. On the contrary it had provided a sure base from which the educational opportunities arising as the work progressed were taken up and used to advantage while the pace and thrust of the work were maintained.

In these examples of good practice in primary schools the overriding characteristic is that of agreed, clear aims and purposeful teaching.

Analysis

It is worth analysing the characteristics that HMI identifies as typifying good practice. Significantly, it highlights the importance of the wider learning environment in which individual classrooms, children and teachers are operating. While one might identify an oasis of good practice in an individual classroom, the impact is seriously limited if the values and practices are not shared among the wider school community. For children this would create a sense of unease and confusion and, as discussed earlier, a sense of security and well-being is vital for learning to be effective.

Analysing the HMI extract above brings out five key elements of effective practice that relate to classroom atmosphere and ethos. These are:

- informality;
- clear communication which is two way;
- knowledge of children's backgrounds and abilities;
- teacher commitment;
- agreed shared aims for learning.

This extract was written in 1987, immediately prior to the introduction of the National Curriculum. One might question whether the good practice identified during the 1980s was thwarted by the introduction of a standards-driven agenda which focused on the formal outcomes of an academic and skills-focused curriculum. English (2005) outlines the key strands in this debate, and notes the huge changes that were brought about, with the National Curriculum prescribing what should be taught, and then the Literacy and Numeracy Strategies (DfES, 1998, 1999) dictating how this content should be delivered. We are perhaps at a seminal moment now with the introduction of the Primary Strategy (DfES, 2003b) providing for scope and flexibility in the *what* and the *how* of the curriculum.

Teachers should seize this opportunity to reflect on their practice and on how they can create a learning environment that fosters the process of learning through effective, affective relationships. The guidance for inspectors cited in the preparatory reading, although published some 16 years after the extract above, dictates what should be used as evidence to judge effective teaching. Perhaps you can still see the importance of classroom atmosphere in the following statement about what *very good* teaching and learning look like:

> … all pupils are engrossed in their work and make considerably better progress than might be expected. Achievement is high. Teaching is stimulating, enthusiastic and consistently challenging, stemming from expert knowledge of the curriculum, how to teach it and how pupils learn. There are excellent relationships in the classroom. Teaching methods are well selected and time issued very productively for whole-class, independent and collaborative work. Activities and demands are matched sensitively to pupils' needs. Well directed teaching assistants reinforce and support learning very effectively. (OFSTED, 2003a, Table 10)

Practical implications and activities

The OFSTED criteria have been synthesised for the purposes of this activity:

- pupil achievement;
- teaching strategies;
- teacher subject knowledge;
- classroom relationships;
- pupil activities;
- classroom assistants.

1. Recall a lesson you have taught or observed that you feel was successful. Comment on it with reference to each of the bullet points above.

2. Now reflect on an unsuccessful lesson. Using the bullet points above, can you identify what elements of the lesson were contributing to it being unsuccessful? What changes would you make?

3. Which of these relate to the classroom atmosphere? Is it possible to segment these or are they interrelated?

How?

Before you read the following extract, read:

- Pollard, A (2005) *Reflective teaching*, 2nd edition, Chapter 6. London: Continuum.

In this chapter Pollard discusses the classroom atmosphere and relationships from the perspectives of those involved.

Extract: DfES (2004c) *Behaviour in the classroom: A course for newly qualified teachers.* **www.standards.dfes.gov.uk (accessed July 2005).**

OHT 2.1
Aims of the session

Session Two will explore:

- how expectations about behaviour are set
- using expectations in the classroom
- a solution-focused strategy for developing expectations
- how to change and develop expectations
- creating a positive learning environment:
  - physical
  - emotional

and will continue to build on:

- a proactive checklist for positive behaviour management

OHT 2.2
Why are expectations important?
- Children and adults need to know what is expected of them if they are to be successful
- Clarifying expectations helps to create a positive atmosphere by emphasising what is wanted and valued
- Stating specific expectations offers a framework for explicitly identifying the behaviours you need to teach so that all children have the opportunity to succeed

Handout 2.1

Understanding expectations

What do we mean by the term 'expectations'?	
•	
List below some examples of expectations that are evident in your own classroom	Where does each of these expectations come from?
•	•
•	•
•	•
•	•
•	•
How do your children know that these expectations exist?	
•	
•	
•	

OHT 2.3

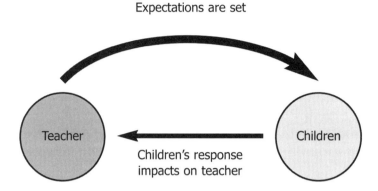

Expectations are set

Teacher

Children

Children's response
impacts on teacher

A solution-focused strategy for developing expectations in my classroom

HANDOUT 2.2
To what extent are my expectations being met?

Part 1
The first part of this activity is done individually. You do not need to share your personal information.

Think about your own class and classroom and how satisfied you feel at present about the degree to which you are achieving what you want in terms of a well-managed classroom environment. Look at the descriptors at each end of the scale below and put a mark to indicate where you feel you are now.

0 ——————————————————————————————————— 10

*I feel I have not helped children
understand my expectations about
their behaviour for learning at all*

*I feel I have helped children
understand my expectations
about their behaviour for learning
very successfully*

Now put a mark on the scale at the point where you would like to be by the end of this course (or at a time suggested by the course leader).

Part 2
Now work with a partner. You do not have to say where you have rated yourself now or what rating you have set yourself.

First, with your partner explore exactly what it is that you are already doing to ensure that you are at the point where you have placed yourself (i.e. generate a list of successful strategies which you are using already). Then talk to your partner about what will be happening in your classroom when you reach the point you have chosen as where you would like to get to.

OHT 2.5
Setting and changing expectations
• Explicit description of the behaviour you require

- Clarity: use precise language
- Involvement of children
- Involve support from colleagues as necessary

OHT 2.6
Reviewing expectations
- Consider how you will monitor the success of your expectations
- How frequently will you review what is happening in the classroom?
- How will you involve the children and others?
- How will you celebrate success?
- How will you deal with any revisions?

OHT 2.7
Classroom organisation for positive behaviour: physical

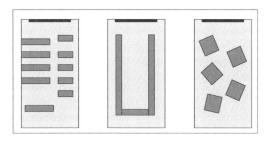

Handout 2.4
Classroom environment checklist

This checklist is designed to help you examine the context in which behaviour occurs. Only those statements which apply to your setting need to be considered. Many of the questions could be answered during a tour of the setting.

	Definitely	Mostly	Partly	Not at all
The classroom is attractive and inviting				
Adequate lighting				
Appropriate temperature and ventilation				
Acoustics adequate				
Furniture arranged to best effect				
There is a seating plan which is known by the children				
Clearly defined pathways with sufficient space for children to move freely between activities				
Routines foster a calm and positive atmosphere				
Routines encourage children to make choices				
Chalk board, whiteboard, etc. easily seen				
Quiet area available				
Differing learning areas are clearly delineated				
Room organisation meets differing curriculum needs				
Materials easily accessible and visibly labelled to support children's independent learning				
Materials/resources match the learning styles of a wide range of individuals				
Provision and organisation of materials/activities support the development of social, emotional and behavioural skills				

OHT 2.8

Classroom organisation for positive behaviour: emotional

Children need to feel:

- safe
- welcome
- valued
- supported
- motivated

Handout 2.5

A proactive checklist to promote positive behaviour in my classroom: sections 2 and 3

2. *My expectations of the children's behaviour*

- What do I expect them to be doing at each stage of the session/lesson?
- How will I teach these expectations?
- How can I build this teaching into my curriculum planning?
- How can I involve my children in setting expectations for themselves?
- How can I reinforce the expectations over time?

3. *Planning the classroom environment*

- How will I physically organise the learning environment to promote positive behaviour?
- How will I ensure that children feel emotionally safe and nurtured in my classroom?

Analysis

Student teachers who find classroom life challenging can easily slip into a negative *blame* spiral, which means they find it difficult to see a positive way forward. The Primary National Strategy team adopts a proactive and forward-looking approach to supporting new teachers in the classroom. The illustrative materials above are extracts from an online course on behaviour management. They promote a *solution-focused* approach, to support teachers in taking positive steps in their own classrooms. The focus on behaviour management is driven by surveys of NQTs (TTA, 2005), which support claims that this group of teachers feels ill prepared by their initial training for this area of their work. Behaviour management will be discussed at greater length in Chapters 8 and 9.

For the purposes of this chapter it is useful to explore the link between classroom climate and behaviour and how the two are interdependent, with a particular focus on clear communication being at the heart of good practice. Pollard (2005) identifies the need for a *working consensus* to exist between all sharing the classroom space, including children, support staff and teachers. This consensus is based upon a shared understanding of expectations and a willingness to acknowledge the needs of others. If we then review the course materials above it is clear that the basis is upon the use of clear communication to outline expectations. While it is evident that the children are involved in the process of outlining expectations (OHT in extract 2.3 above), reciprocity is not as strongly stressed as one might expect. There seems to be an over-emphasis upon the teacher having a clear idea of his/her own working requirements, and the focus of the training programme then becomes *how to get the children to behave as the teacher wants* rather than being a negotiation about how all involved are going to work in the shared learning space that is the classroom or school. Pollard (2005) claims that children expect the teacher to lead in this process and will respond positively so long as their perception is one of fair treatment.

In this context it is interesting to review how teachers can change expectations (see OHT 2.5 in extract above). Clarity of explanation and the involvement of the children will help them to understand the justification for and equity of the changes being implemented.

Practical implications and applications

Using the *classroom environment checklist*, audit a classroom in which you have worked or are working.

1. What changes do you need to implement?
2. What process will you go through to effect these changes?

Explore the extent to which children are involved in the creation of your positive classroom environment.

Summary

In this chapter you have been challenged to explore how relationships and preferred teaching styles might cause a sense of tension and stress for teachers as they reflect upon their dual role as instructor and carer. It is important to think about the values underpinning these reflections as they will influence how you seek to resolve your identity in the classroom and with the children you teach. In order to seek to achieve the positive learning environment, it is useful to look at the work of Rogers (1969), who focuses upon classroom interactions that demonstrate understanding and giving. These require teachers to have:

- open-mindedness;
- commitment;
- responsibility.

This chapter opened with an acknowledgement of the importance of teachers' own perspectives in developing their work in the classroom. Pollard (2005, p122) sums this up by noting that:

> … we too [teachers] need to feel the benefit of a degree of acceptance, genuineness and empathy.

As a new teacher entering the profession it is thus important that you take opportunities to participate in consultation, whether this be formally through unions or government channels or informally in staff-room conversation. As education moves to a point of massive change (*Every Child Matters*, Workforce Reform, etc.) it will be increasingly important to feel that teachers' voices are listened to and are used to effect change for the good of all in schools. Multidisciplinary teams working in schools will have a range of views and expertise, so genuine sharing and reciprocity of ideas will become increasingly important.

Further reading

Blandford, S (2005) *Sonia Blandford's masterclass*. London: Sage.

English, E and Newton, L (2005) *Professional studies in the primary school*. London: David Fulton.

Kyriacou, C (1991) *Essential teaching skills*. Cheltenham: StanleyThornes.

OFSTED (2003) *Inspecting schools: handbook for inspecting nursery and primary schools*. London: HMSO.

Pollard, A (2005) *Reflective teaching*, 2nd edition. London: Continuum.

7 Classroom interaction and management

By the end of this chapter you should have:

- further considered **why** classroom management and interaction are dependent on relationships between child and teacher;
- critically evaluated **what** elements of a teacher's manner, persona and style might be important influencing factors in classroom management;
- analysed **how** your own developing understanding of yourself as a teacher provides a foundation from which to consider how you might manage the learning interactions in your classroom.

Linking your learning

- Jacques, K and Hyland, R (2003) *Achieving QTS. Professional studies: primary phase*, Chapter 8. Exeter: Learning Matters.

Professional Standards for QTS
1.3, 2.7, 3.3.1, 3.3.7, 3.3.8, 3.3.9

Introduction

This chapter should be read in conjunction with the preceding and following chapters. While exploring the themes around classroom interactions the focus is on the practicalities of the complex world that is a primary classroom. If anything, this chapter should leave you in no doubt that primary teachers are multidimensional, highly skilled and very talented individuals. Primary classrooms, in which they operate, are a complex web of interrelationships, personalities and characters. The ability to manage interactions in such an environment is worthy of considerable respect. Bundy's chapter, cited above, provides you with an introduction to the issues of which you, as a new teacher, need to be aware. He moves from the sophisticated to the simple, exploring issues on how to define your expectations right down to the stopping strategy that you might choose to employ.

As primary classrooms move to a period of change, with more curriculum flexibility and autonomy for teachers (DfES, 2003b), and a larger and multi-skilled workforce operating in schools, it will be ever more important that you as a teacher are able to reflect on what you are doing and why you are doing it that way. The process of articulating this brings clarity and shared understanding for all involved.

As you read through this chapter, you are asked to reflect on these two underpinning questions:

1. How does the manner and style you adopt in the classroom support you to be in role as teacher?

2. In what ways do the *Standards for Qualified Teacher Status* (TTA, 2003c) support you in adopting a management style that reflects your own values and views of education?

Why?

Before you read the following extracts, read:

- Barnes, D (2002) 'Knowledge, communication and learning', in Pollard, A (ed) *Reading for reflective teaching*. London: Continuum.
- Edwards, D and Mercer, N (2002) 'Classroom discourse and learning', in Pollard, A (ed) *Reading for reflective teaching*. London: Continuum.

The following two short extracts provide thought-provoking discussions on elements of culture and communication in classroom interactions.

Extract: Arthur, J, Davison, J and Lewis, M (2005) *Professional Values and Practice*, pp42–45. London: RoutledgeFalmer.

The Hay McBer study is concerned with elucidating three aspects of effective teaching: professional characteristics, teaching skills and classroom climate. We will look briefly at professional characteristics and classroom climate. The relevance of these to the issues explored in this chapter is clear from the study's opening remarks:

> The three factors are different in nature. Two of them – professional characteristics and teaching skills – are factors which relate to what a teacher brings to the job. The professional characteristics are the ongoing patterns of behaviour that combine to drive the things we typically do. Amongst those things are the "micro-behaviours" covered by teaching skills. Whilst teaching skills can be learned, sustaining these behaviours over the course of a career will depend on the deeper seated nature of professional characteristics. Classroom climate, on the other hand, is an output measure. It allows teachers to understand how the pupils in their class feel about nine dimensions of climate created by the teacher that influence their motivation to learn. (Hay McBer, 2000: 7)

We can align 'what a teacher brings to the job' – 'professional characteristics' – with QTS Standard 1.3's requirement for teachers to *demonstrate* certain characteristics; and we can align 'dimensions of climate created by the teacher' – 'classroom climate' – with the other key verb in the Standard: *promote*.

Hay McBer identifies 15 'professional characteristics' divided into five groups. The language is rather different from that used in *Qualifying to Teach* but, more importantly, the list offers a more systematic *conceptualisation* of a wider range of essential attributes, each of which carries with it certain assumptions about Professional Values and Practices. We should note that this categorization of characteristics includes some (like 'Flexibility' and 'Teamworking') which are addressed or implied in various QTS Standards. Nevertheless, it is valuable to have this holistic perspective to complement the way the Standards deal separately with some of these issues.

Professional Characteristics (Hay McBer, 2000: 21–26)

Professionalism	Challenge and support	A commitment to do everything possible for each pupil and enable all pupils to be successful.
	Confidence	The belief in one's ability to be effective and to take on challenges.
	Creating trust	Being consistent and fair. Keeping one's word.
	Respect for others	The underlying belief that individuals matter and deserve respect.
Thinking	Analytical thinking	The ability to think logically, break things down, and recognise cause and effect.
	Conceptual thinking	The ability to see patterns and links, even when there is a lot of detail.
Planning and Setting Expectations	Drive for improvement	Relentless energy for setting and meeting challenging targets for pupils and the school.
	Information seeking	A drive to find out more and get to the heart of things; intellectual curiosity.
	Initiative	The drive to act now and pre-empt events.
Leading	Flexibility	The ability and willingness to adapt to the needs of a situation and change tactics.
	Holding people accountable	The drive and ability to set clear expectations and parameters and to hold others accountable for performance.
	Managing pupils	The drive and the ability to provide clear direction to pupils, and to enthuse and motivate them.
	Passion for learning	The drive and an ability to support pupils in their learning, and to help them become confident and independent learners.
Relating to Others	Impact and influence	The ability and the drive to produce positive outcomes by impressing and influencing others.
	Teamworking	The ability to work with others to achieve shared goals.
	Understanding others	The drive and ability to understand others, and why they behave as they do.

We suggest that this is a useful checklist when undertaking lesson observations. What examples of these characteristics can you see in observed lessons? What specific teaching and learning strategies and events provide *evidence* of them in operation? Look back at 'A Lesson Observed' and see whether you can match features which were described there to some of these more generically expressed characteristics.

Going a little further, consider for a moment the two aspects of 'Thinking' in the Hay McBer list: 'analytical' – breaking things down, and 'conceptual' – seeing patterns and links. Taking a particular topic which would form the substance of one lesson, how would you plan for both of these with, say, a Year 7 class?

One further practical exercise, this time relating to 'flexibility', is: using an occasion from your own teaching experience when you were aware that you either *did* or *did not* 'adapt to the needs of a situation and change tactics', why did you decide the way you did, and what were the consequences? Would you, with hindsight, make a different decision now, in order to achieve a different outcome in terms of learners' engagement or achievement?

Research perspective 2: classroom climate

The Hay McBer study offers nine dimensions of classroom climate, defining it as:

> the collective perceptions by pupils of what it feels like to be a pupil in any particular teacher's classroom, where those perceptions influence every student's motivation to learn and perform to the best of his or her ability. The dimensions are:

Clarity	around the purpose of each lesson. How each lesson relates to the broader subject, as well as clarity regarding the aims and objectives of the school.
Order	within the classroom, where discipline, order and civilised behaviour are maintained.
A clear set of standards	as to how pupils should behave and what each pupil should do and try to achieve, with a clear focus on higher rather than minimum standards.
Fairness	the degree to which there is an absence of favouritism, and a consistent link between rewards in the classroom and actual performance.
Participation	the opportunity for pupils to participate actively in the class by discussion, questioning, giving out materials and other similar activities.
Support	feeling emotionally supported in the classroom, so that pupils are willing to try new things and learn from mistakes.
Safety	the degree to which the classroom is a safe place, where pupils are not at risk from emotional or physical bullying, or other fear-arousing factors.
Interest	the feeling that the classroom is an interesting and exciting place to be, where pupils feel stimulated to learn.
Environment	the feeling that the classroom is a comfortable, well-organised, clean and attractive physical environment.

(Hay McBer (2000) *Classroom climate*, pp27–28)

We might, perhaps, add one more dimension. It is certainly the case that if you ask children why some teachers make lessons interesting and motivating, time and time again they will put 'fun' at the top of the list. This is, however, a slightly risky concept, and it is easy to see why it has not found its way into a report like the Hay McBer study. We would propose, though, that the descriptor for 'Interest' should perhaps be: 'the feeling that the classroom is an interesting, exciting *and enjoyable* place to be …', and that somewhere in any list of professional characteristics should be included: 'a sense of humour'. The Year 5 primary class's wall display list of values included 'Ability to play' and 'Enjoyment'.

Analysis

The above extract from Arthur *et al.* (2005) draws on the credible research work of Hay McBer (2000) and clearly links professional characteristics to the ability to *produce* a certain type of classroom climate. Itemising the attributes of the classroom climate perhaps provides a distancing framework through which reflective teachers can analyse their own style of management and resulting organisation.

Personal response and reflections

1. Reflecting on your last placement or a classroom you know well, how far did the management and interactions demonstrate:

   - clarity;
   - order;
   - a clear set of standards;
   - fairness;
   - participation;
   - support;
   - safety;
   - interest;
   - environment.

2. To what extent does there need to be a balance of attributes to bring about successful learning interaction and management?

Barnes (2002) suggests that the balance and emphasis will shift, not according to the skills and characteristics of the teacher, as suggested by Arthur et al. (2005), but in response to the teacher's conception of knowledge and learning. A teacher who views knowledge as a public discipline will use interactions that focus on transmission, assessment and presentation. In contrast, the teacher who holds that knowledge is a fluid act of interpretation will use interactions that support negotiation, collaboration and context (Barnes, 2002).

It is interesting to overlay the Hay McBer (2000) professional characteristics with Barnes's two views on the nature of knowledge. Arthur et al. (2005) do attempt to distinguish between the innate qualities a teacher brings to the job and those skills that can be acquired through training. This leads one to question the extent to which teachers are somehow preconditioned to interact and manage in a particular way that is directly dependent on the professional characteristics they bring to the class-room. Arthur et al. (2005) explore how this is interpreted in the teacher training standards (TTA, 2003c), and it is possible to detect a shift in the perception of knowledge that underpins these standards. Hayes (1997), writing about the early versions of the TTA competencies (DfE circular 14/93), lists issues about the model of training being developed and notes that *at the heart of these concerns is a belief that teaching cannot be deconstructed into a number of discrete and separately identifiable parts*

(1997, p166). Today, although still open to some criticism, there is a more holistic emphasis on teacher development and the prioritising of *professional values and practice* (TTA, 2003c). It could be seen that this development in the standards reflects less of an emphasis on knowledge as a discrete public discipline, and that they now represent more of an attempt to promote a process-based curriculum.

What?

Before you read the following extract, read:

- Kyriacou, C (1991) *Essential teaching skills*, Chapter 5. Cheltenham: StanleyThornes.

This chapter provides a very practical consideration of issues around classroom climate.

Extract: Pollard, A and Tann, S (1993) *Reflective Teaching in the Primary School. A handbook for the classroom*, 2nd edition, pp207–209. London: Cassell.

1.1 'Withitness'

'Withitness' is a term coined by Kounin (1970) to describe the capacity to be aware of the wide variety of things which are simultaneously going on in a classroom. This is a constant challenge for any teacher and can be a particular strain for a new teacher until this skill is acquired.

Teachers who are 'with it' are said to 'have eyes in the back of their head'. They are able to anticipate and to see where help is needed. They are able to nip trouble in the bud. They are skilful at scanning the class while helping individuals and they position themselves accordingly. They are alert; they can pre-empt disturbance; and they can act fast. They can sense the way a class is responding and can act to maintain a positive atmosphere.

1.2 'Overlapping'

This is another of Kounin's terms and describes the skill of being able to do more than one thing at the same time. This can be related to withitness if, for example, a problem emerges concerning occasions when giving sustained help to a particular child results in relatively neglecting the rest of the class. In addition, overlapping is also an important and separate skill in its own right. Most teachers work under such pressure that they have to think about and do more than one thing at a time. Decisions have to be made very rapidly. Jackson (1968) calculated that over a thousand interpersonal exchanges a day typically take place between each teacher and the children in their care. For these reasons, reflecting, anticipating and making rapid judgements are very much a necessary part of any teacher's skills.

1.3 Pacing

Pacing a teaching-learning session is another important skill. It involves making appropriate judgements about the timing and phasing of the various activities and parts of a session and then taking suitable actions. At the simplest level, there is the practical judgement to be made at the end of a session about when to switch into a 'tidying up phase' – it is very easy to get involved in activities, forget about the clock and suddenly to find that it is playtime. More complex educational judgements are necessary in relation to learning activities and the various phases of a typical session. For instance, the activities have to be introduced: this is often an initial 'motivational phase' where the children's interest is stimulated. This motivation also has to be maintained. Sessions then often enter an 'incubation and development phase' in which children think about the activities, explore ideas and then tackle tasks. From time to time there may be a need for a 'restructuring phase' where objectives and procedures may need to be clarified further. Finally, there may be a 'review phase' for reinforcing good effort or for reflecting on overall progress.

Judgements about pacing – about when to make a new initiative – depend crucially on being sensitive to how children are responding to activities. If they are immersed and productively engaged then one might decide to extend a phase or run the activity into the next session. If the children seem to be becoming bored, frustrated or listless then it is usually wise to retain the initiative, to restructure or review the activity or to move on to something new. If the children are becoming too 'high', excited and distracted, then it may be useful to review and maybe redirect them into an activity which calms them down by rechannelling their energies.

1.4 Self-presentation
The last of the four management skills which we have identified is self-presentation, for how to 'present' oneself to children is also a matter for skill and judgement. Teachers who are able to project themselves so that children expect them to be 'in charge' have a valuable ability. There is a very large element of self-confidence in this, and student teachers, in particular, may sometimes find it difficult to enact the change from the student role to the teacher role. Perhaps this is not surprising, for a huge change in rights and responsibilities is involved. The first essential, then, is to believe in oneself as a teacher.

A second range of issues concerned with self-presentatlon is more skill-based. Here non-verbal cues are important. Self-presentation relates to such things as gesture, posture, movement, position in the room, facial expression, etc. These will be actively interpreted by children. The intended impression might be one of sureness, of confidence and competence. The reflective teacher will need to consider how non-verbal cues can help to convey such attributes.

A further very important skill is voice control. A teacher's use of voice can be highly sophisticated and effective. Changing the pitch, volume, projection and the intensity of meaning can communicate different aspects about self. If anyone's voice is to be used in this way it will require some training and time to develop. Teachers, like singers and actors, can learn to use their diaphragm to project a 'chest voice', to breathe more deeply and speak more slowly so that their voice and their message is carried more effectively. Developing voice control is also an important asset in telling and reading stories, which may involve having to present many different characters. In the first instance it may be a good idea to try out different 'voices' – privately, and far enough away from others that a 'big' voice does not disturb anyone else! Although tape-recorders never seem flattering, recording a practice story-telling can be a useful way of seeing how much appropriate voice variety is developing.

A fourth and more general area of skill which is involved in how teachers present and project themselves is that of 'acting' – as though on a stage. In this sense it is the ability to convey what we mean by 'being a teacher', so that expectations are clear and relationships can be negotiated.

Acting is also an enormous strength for teachers for one other particular reason. When one is acting one is partially detached from the role. It is possible to observe oneself, to analyse, reflect and plan. Acting, in other words, is controlled behaviour which is partially distanced from self. In the situations of vulnerability which sometimes arise in classrooms this can be a great asset.

The skills which we have been reviewing above need to be put in a context. They are simply skills and have no substantive content or merit in their own right. A self-confident performer who lacks purpose and gets practical matters wrong (for example has ill-defined objectives, mixes up children's names, plans sessions badly, loses books, acts unfairly, etc.) will not be able to manage a class. A teacher has to be competent as well as skilled and must understand the ends of education as well as the means.

Analysis

Pollard and Tann take some of the issues discussed in the previous section and begin to ground them in the reality of classroom management. The chapter from Kyriacou, cited above, challenges trainee teachers to explore key questions concerning their own management style. Both excerpts highlight the complex and multidimensional nature of classroom interaction and management.

Kounin (1970) refers to teachers needing the skills of *withitness* and *overlapping*. These refer to the physical ability to be aware of a range of activities, people and learning at any one time, and the use of professional intuition to make quick decisions to assist the progress of learning in the classroom. Pollard and Tann stress that these skills can be particularly demanding for the new teacher. Beginning teachers need to invest time observing experienced practitioners at work, and then be supported by a mentor to deconstruct the multilayered nature of what they are seeing. This is particularly important if they are observing very effective practice, as the teacher will make seamless transitions from one interaction to the next, and be reflecting and making judgements intuitively – all of which can mask the complexity of the learning management.

Pace and timing are two of the key ingredients of successful classroom management and interaction. Government strategies to support literacy and numeracy (DfES, 1998, 1999) in the primary sector really brought pace to the fore in lesson planning and management. Lesson structures were promoted that focused on pacey delivery and quick transitions to compartmentalised segments of lessons. This was enshrined as good practice by making it a requirement that new teachers must teach the strategies to qualify (TTA, 2003c, 3.3.2b). Qualified teachers are judged by OFSTED on whether they make effective use of time (OFSTED, 2003a). It is important, however, to ensure that effective use of time does not always equate to speed and a quick pace; increasing the *wait* time for a response to a question can provide for a more comfortable working environment and facilitate thoughtful reflection.

Personal presentation is identified as a crucial factor in classroom management and interaction (Pollard and Tann, 1993). It is as much about believing yourself to be in role as teacher as what you wear and how you address the children. Hughes (2002) gives various reasons for thinking about your own dress code: respect, credibility, acceptance and authority. Most importantly, she says, teachers are *acting as a role model for children, so you need to look professional, proud, dedicated, responsible and appreciated* (Hughes, 2002, p72). Personal presentation also includes body language, and voice which, as Griffiths notes, *is a remarkable instrument, capable of infinite variation which allows it to convey a wide range of thoughts, ideas and feelings* (Griffiths, 2000, p141). It is this ability to convey *hidden* values, attitudes and views that teachers must consider when reflecting on how they are to manage and interact in their classroom. This is explored further in response to the extract from Grossman, below.

How?

Before you read the following extract, read:

- Hughes, P (2000) *Principles of primary education study guide*, 2nd edition, Chapter 7. London: David Fulton.

This chapter provides a practical overview of the key considerations.

Extract: Grossman, H (2004) *Classroom Behaviour Management for Diverse and Inclusive Schools*, 3rd edition, pp28–30. Oxford: Rowan and Littlefield.

Being genuine
Almost everyone responds to a person who is genuine. Teachers are genuine when their words and actions express their true feelings and opinions. And when teachers are genuine, their students know they can trust what the teacher tells them.

Teachers have two basic reasons for not always being genuine. They may not be able to admit to themselves that they have certain feelings, or they may not be able to express their feelings to the students. Certain teachers may hide their positive feelings from their students, but more often teachers are uncomfortable about expressing or even feeling their negative emotions.

If your answers to the self-quiz on communication with students suggest that you might have difficulty being genuine with them, Chernow and Chernow (203) suggest that accepting the following three basic truths will help you be more honest:

Self-quiz: working with low achievers
Your answers to the following questions about low achievers will help you evaluate how fair you are being in your work with them. Do you:

Call on low achievers less frequently to answer questions or demonstrate something?

Wait less time for them to answer?

Give them less encouragement or assistance after you have called on them?

Praise them for answers that really aren't correct?

Interrupt them when they are reciting?

Maintain less eye contact with them when you are lecturing?

Require less work of them for the same credit?

Seat them far from you?

Self-quiz: communication with students

Do you think you would be able to communicate the following to your students in an appropriate way?

Disapproval of a student's behavior

Anger at the way the student relates to the opposite gender

Anger at the way the student treats you

Disappointment that the student didn't keep a promise to you

Mistrust of the student's emotion

Disbelief in what the student says

Which of the following do you think you would have trouble admitting even to yourself?

Dislike for a student as a person

Discomfort with a student's disability

Preconceived notions about the student's honesty, motivation, potential, and so on, based on the student's gender, ethnic group, or socioeconomic background

Disappointment that the student doesn't appear to like you despite your efforts

1. In the natural course of events, students will sometimes make you uncomfortable, angry, and even furious.
2. You are entitled to have these feelings without also experiencing guilt or shame, because they are natural.
3. You are entitled to express your feelings as long as you do so in a way that doesn't harm your students.

To constantly 'stuff your feelings' – try to act as if nothing bothers you – can quickly lead to teacher burnout. The goal here is to express your real feelings in ways that help, not harm, your students. For example, suppose you are explaining to Tom why he shouldn't have picked on a younger student during recess. But instead of listening to you, Tom is looking around the yard and making it clear that he has no interest in what you're saying. You tell him that he is not listening, but he keeps looking around. You feel frustrated and more than a little upset. You tell yourself that he is just being defensive, that he is not purposely trying to get you angry. But that doesn't change your feelings, and a rage starts building inside of you. You recall that the last time you felt like this you walked away rather than express your feelings, but that only made you angrier because it seemed like that was what Tom wanted. Just remembering this makes you even angrier now. What should you do?

First, you need not feel guilty or think you are a poor teacher for being angry. Most people would get angry in that situation. Second, you should not try to mask your feelings behind a smile and walk away. Instead, tell Tom how you feel but in a way that does not attack him personally. You can do this by focusing on his behavior, not on him as a person.

'Tom, I'm getting angry. I feel you're not paying attention to what I'm saying, and that upsets me.' This would be one acceptable way of expressing your feelings. Another good way would be to say, 'Tom, when I see you looking everywhere but at me when I'm trying to tell you something important, it seems like you're not listening and don't care. That upsets me.' Then a good follow-up, after expressing your feelings, is to set clear expectations for future behavior: 'I'd like you to listen when I talk to you so we can get back to the business of you being a good student and me doing my job, too.' Comments like 'What's the matter with you, didn't anyone ever teach you to look at people when they talk to you?' and 'Look at me when I'm talking to you' are two inappropriate ways of expressing yourself because they belittle Tom as a person.

By the way, failure to maintain eye contact is not always a sign of disrespect. As you will see in chapter 5, unlike students from European backgrounds who are taught to look at adults when they are being spoken to, students from African and Hispanic backgrounds are brought up to look away when they are being reprimanded.

Being friendly

Friendly teachers are effective managers. They are open, approachable, and available rather than closed, distant, and aloof. They are also interested in their students as people and are willing to listen to things that aren't directly related to their students' education. In turn, they reveal their interests and the kind of people they are by sharing their feelings, values, and opinions. This makes them 'come alive' for their students. Although no teacher can actually be a friend of thirty students or six classes of thirty students, teachers can be friendly.

A word of caution is in order. Students are not all equally responsive to their teachers' friendly overtures. Some students, particularly from certain Asian Pacific Island groups, are used to and prefer more formal relationships with their teachers. Some students with emotional problems are threatened by close relationships (see chapter 13). Therefore, if your attempts to be friendly with students are not accepted, it may be wiser to ask yourself why and back off rather than redouble your efforts.

There are two types of friendly teachers, one effective, the other ineffective (208). The first develop friendly relationships with students based on strength, respect, and trust while they maintain their role as the person in charge. The second type, motivated by a need to be accepted by students in order to build up their own self-esteem, reject taking charge and choose a weak role for themselves. The first type of friendly relationship with students is positive; the second is destructive and leaves the class without strong leadership.

Analysis

Grossman's work is primarily aimed at the US audience and, as a result, some of the style and terminology might be unfamiliar. But the honest openness about some of the sensitive issues around classroom interactions makes for refreshing reading. Underpinning Grossman's advice to teachers as they manage and interact in their classrooms is the need for them to be genuine in all that they do.

Personal response and reflection

Hughes (2002, pp77–78) lists the following theoretical bases for management of children:

- the counselling approach;
- the democratic approach;
- the behavioural approach;
- the research-based empirical approach;
- the cognitive approach;
- the ecological and ecosystemic approach;
- the assertive discipline approach.

1. Reflecting on classrooms in which you have some management responsibility, where have you felt most able to be *genuine* with the children?

2. Have you developed your pedagogy and management style in a way that reflects a balance of the above?

Grossman's other key piece of advice is to be *friendly* towards the children with whom you are interacting. The issues surrounding the tensions within a friendly professional relationship were discussed in the previous chapter, but it is interesting to note Grossman's bold statement that *friendly teachers are effective managers* (2004, p30) – although not when the teacher's own insecurities motivate them to desire the affection of the children. Oldham (2005) reinforces Grossman's statement by noting that teachers *cannot afford to obtain [an orderly classroom] at the expense of mutually respectful relationships with pupils* (p41).

In his discussion Grossman does allude to a range of culturally influenced responses to teacher interactions. Children from within particular communities may have expectations of the role of the teacher, or accepted ways of demonstrating respect, that may be at odds with the style of management and interaction that is being promoted by the teacher. To this end it is essential that teachers take time to know and understand cultural nuances and expectations, without falling in danger of stereotyping. The QTS standards (TTA, 2003c) make provision for this element of teacher development – however it is more likely that this is a type of knowledge and understanding that will develop in a situation-specific context. As Oldham (2005) observes, relationships, boundaries and interactions in the classroom are in a constant state of flux and negotiation.

Practical implications and activities

Hughes (2002, pp72–73) provides an invaluable checklist against which you can consider some practical implications for your interactions and management style.

- Dress appropriately.
- Value yourself.
- Share yourself.
- Keep a sense of humour.
- Remember you're a learner too.
- Be tough.
- Reward effort.
- See the invisible children.

1. Taking a day or a week from a previous school placement, reflect on how far you were able to demonstrate or model the points above. If you were to turn the clock back, what concrete actions could you have taken to ensure you made a positive response to Hughes' list?

2. Share your thoughts with a peer or colleague.

Summary

This chapter has focused very much on you as the teacher, and on how your presence, manner and personality can influence the interactions you have with children. It is impossible to consider your management style in isolation as it will be influenced and shaped by your own understanding of the nature of education and the resulting values that will emerge. But the tensions and issues that emerge are ones to be explored rather than, as Grossman (2004) observes, *to be bottled up*. As noted earlier in this book, it is an exciting time to be in education as the school curriculum is changing. *Excellence and Enjoyment* (DfES, 2003b) gives teachers and schools the opportunity to be selective, creative and innovative in the way they deliver the curriculum. One strand that has emerged in this chapter is that when teachers have the opportunity to enjoy and be stimulated by their work they feel more able to express confidence in their relationships and classroom management. Perhaps these times of change offer that exciting prospect?

Further Reading

Blandford, S (2004) *School Discipline Manual*. London: Pearson.
Hay McBer, D (2000) *Research into Teacher Effectiveness: A Model of Teacher Effectiveness*. Report to the DfEE, June 2000. London: DfEE.
Herne, S, Jessel, J and Griffiths, J (2000) *Study to Teach*. London: Routledge.
TTA (2003c) *Qualifying to Teach*. London: HMSO.

8 Managing challenging behaviour

By the end of this chapter you should have:

- further considered **why** effective learning leads to positive behaviour;
- critically evaluated **what** role the school community ethos and partnership with parents plays in preventing and minimising incidents of challenging behaviour;
- analysed **how** your own developing pedagogy and values of education provide a foundation for reflection as you manage incidents of challenging behaviour.

Linking your learning

- Jacques, K and Hyland, R (2003) *Achieving QTS. Professional studies: primary phase*, Chapter 9. Exeter: Learning Matters.

Professional Standards for QTS
2.7, 3.3.9

Introduction

The overriding message in all contemporary literature about behaviour management is that serious disruptive behaviour is extremely rare (for example, Hayes, 2004, Grossman, 2004, OFSTED, 2005b). However, it remains an area that is of considerable concern to new teachers (TTA, 2005). The level of resourcing for materials that support teachers in behaviour management perhaps reflects this concern, rather than the reality of the issue in schools. However, the research and the materials that are being funded by government agencies are promoting a line that it is to be welcomed. Projects such as the Evidence for Policy and Practice Information (EPPI) systematic review of how theories explain learning behaviour in school contexts, and the Behaviour4Learning's ITT Professional Resource Network (IPRN), are grounded in the belief that behaviour and learning are inseparable. They challenge the notion that *behaviour management [is] solely concerned with establishing control over disruptive pupils* (Powell and Tod, 2004).

This chapter concludes Section 2, and should be read in conjunction with Chapters 4 to 7. The issues discussed are relevant to the management of challenging behaviour in the classroom. There is a plethora of contemporary literature in this field – much of it attempting to appeal to the desire for *quick tips* to remedy incidents of challenging behaviour. This chapter does not follow that line – the underlying beliefs promoted support the premise that effective teaching and management will result in positive behaviour patterns.

As you work through this chapter, it will be useful to think about the following two questions:

1. What opportunities do behaviour management strategies afford for the child's voice to be heard?

2. How far can you attribute positive behaviour to effective teaching?

Why?

Before you read the following extract, read:

- Blandford, S (2004) *School discipline manual*, Section 3. London: Pearson.

This section is helpful in showing that behaviour management strategies are effective if set within a wider context than just the classroom.

Extract: Powell, S and Tod, J (2004) *Research Evidence in Education in Education Library*, pp11–12. London: EPPI Centre.

Actions and contexts that could promote positive behaviours and decrease negative behaviours

Medium to high weight evidence suggests that practices in relation to promoting good behaviour (QTS S1.3) and managing behaviour (S3.3.9) could be improved by the following:

- promoting mastery orientation rather than performance orientation
- using heterogeneous groupings and facilitative teaching approaches
- promoting on-task verbal interaction between pupils
- working in partnership with pupils in goal-setting so that a shared understanding can be established in relation to anticipating and addressing barriers to learning
- discouraging competitive classroom contexts and encouraging positive inter-personal relationships.

Interpretation of review findings suggest that positive learning behaviours might be also enhanced by:

- teaching that places emphasis on developing effective learning behaviour through subject teaching
- encouraging the application of theory and conceptual frameworks to the task of selecting and evaluating the use of strategies for behaviour management
- redressing the balance between behavioural approaches to behaviour management to include understanding, use and evaluation of cognitive and affective strategies
- enhancing existing assessment procedures to include formative assessment of social, emotional and behavioural indicators of learning
- teaching and assessment that seeks to develop shared understanding of learning behaviour between pupil and teacher coupled with the adoption of assessment practices that value personal achievement
- developing increased integration of the 'social' and 'academic' in recognition of the contribution of personal, social, cultural and family factors on learning and achievement; one way this might be achieved is by the integration of targets from personal, social and health education (PSHE) and citizenship into subject teaching.

Analysis

The text above sets the context for this chapter and, while it is important to support teachers in managing the moment when challenging behaviour is exhibited, it is absolutely central that teachers perceive the wider context and influencing factors that may prevent these behaviour confrontations from coming to fruition. Blandford's (2004) work moves through an exploration of the principles to arrive at practical suggestions. Her work focuses on the notion of community: the community that surrounds the school, and also the community that is the school itself. To an extent, the values and principles of the wider community are reflected in the local school because of the very fact that many of the children will live in the immediate environment. However, in trying to develop a sense of school community and culture it is important to draw on a variety of views to allow for inclusion and ownership.

Personal response and reflection

Reflect on a community to which you belong. How are the beliefs and values evident in the culture that this community has created?

Think about:

- the practices – rites, rituals and ceremonies;
- the communications;
- the physical forms – location, fixtures and fittings;
- the common language.
  (Blandford, 2004)

The notion that a sense of community and its resulting cultural expressions will have a positive impact on classroom behaviour is shared by Powell and Tod (2004). The conceptual framework underpinning their notion of learning behaviours is located within a community context. The social interaction that happens within these communities is the active process by which participants come to own and be part of the culture. This active involvement is highlighted repeatedly in their research, which also suggests that social interaction between children and teachers in schools is crucial for securing positive learning behaviours. Once again, the research seems to be bringing to light the more progressive (McNamara and Moreton, 1997) teaching styles that promote active participation, negotiation and a mutual respect between child and teacher.

The importance of the affective domain, as identified by Blandford (2004) and Powell and Tod (2004), should also be noted, where children are valued and supported in all areas of their development including the social and emotional. This resonates with the ideas discussed in chapter 5, in which research highlighted the necessity of appealing to all areas of the brain in order to foster resilience and an ability to take risks in a safe learning environment.

What?

Before you read the following extract, read:

- Blandford, S (2004) 'Managing positive behaviour', in Clipson-Boyles, S (ed) *Putting research in practice in teaching and learning.* London: David Fulton.

This chapter is significant because it draws on research that set out explicitly to hear the voice of teachers.

Extract: OFSTED (2005b) *Managing Challenging Behaviour*, **pp17–18. London: OFSTED.**

Well-focused pastoral support and guidance
- Support and guidance tend to be good in schools where there is a strong sense of community and the staff regularly celebrate pupils' successes.
- The most effective pastoral support systems are those in which there is careful and regular tracking of pupils' learning and behaviour.
- The role of the tutor in secondary schools and colleges is of great importance in supporting those with the most difficult behaviour. However, the effectiveness of tutor support varies considerably.

What good pastoral systems can do
72. Pastoral systems that are effective for pupils with difficult behaviour are designed to support pupils both with their learning and their behaviour. Where there is a positive ethos in which staff regularly celebrate success, support and guidance tend to be good. A strong sense of community is established. Staff act as excellent role models and they talk with pupils about appropriate ways to behave and respond in difficult situations. Strong relationships are based on mutual respect and staff treat pupils fairly at all times. Teachers know their pupils well and additional support is given to pupils who require it. However, in many of the schools, even where numbers are small, not all staff know all the pupils and this can have a negative effect on the behaviour of the most difficult pupils.
73. In the early years settings and most of the primary schools staff support pupils well. In the secondary schools where support and guidance are good, all staff, from form tutors to senior managers, are involved in the process. In the special schools, PRUs, secure training centres and independent specialist colleges pupils often receive good support from their tutors which has a significant impact in helping them to improve their behaviour.
74. The effectiveness of the tutor system in secondary schools varies considerably. The daily meeting with the form or year tutor can provide an excellent opportunity to reduce tensions, sort out grievances and deal with situations well before they get out of hand. However poorly managed sessions result in quite the opposite. Teachers require training to ensure that tutor time is used to the benefit of all pupils.
75. A good example of a school adapting its system better to support pupils was described by pupils in a school council meeting.

76. Pastoral systems are most effective when there is careful and regular tracking of pupils' social and academic progress. Setting precise targets and rewarding achievement for small improvements is an important part of the process. This happens on a daily basis in many of the special schools, PRUs and secure training centres, but less so in some of the secondary schools. Making time for effective, pastoral support is critical and can lead to the effect resolution of repeated or extended difficult behaviour.

Rewards and celebration

77. Schools which support pupils well are quick to acknowledge and celebrate pupils' achievement and reward systems are applied consistently. Individual rewards help encourage pupils to take responsibility for their own behaviour. However, in some of the schools the focus is on negative behaviour and punishments rather than the rewarding of successes. In some of the general FE colleges achievement may be recognised in lessons but there are few opportunities for the wider sharing of successes.

Responsibilities

78. In many of the schools and units pupils are encouraged to take responsibility for every aspect of school life. Pupils carry out duties in their classroom at an early age and as they become older the responsibilities increase. In these schools teachers listen to pupils and involve them; whole-school decisions, for example, through the school council. Often they develop school and class rules and work alongside staff in setting and reviewing their own targets. 'Circle time' is used well in many of the primary and some of the secondary schools to promote rules and develop strategies to enable pupils to take responsibility. Some of the schools have 'buddy' or peer mentoring systems which support pupils with the most challenging behaviour well. The involvement of pupils in supporting each other could be developed further in many schools.

79. Some of the secondary schools successfully use 'restorative justice' to help pupils take responsibility for their own behaviour. However, a significant number of schools do not encourage pupils to take responsibility or to contribute to decision making processes. Consequently, these schools do not reach those pupils who are more easily disaffected by school.

OFSTED's work has also drawn attention to the importance of a sense of community. Its research findings suggest that, where a school has a developed sense of community, children are also likely to benefit from more developed pastoral and guidance systems. In terms of supporting children who present challenging behaviour, these pastoral support mechanisms provide an opportunity for regular and informed tracking of issues and a place to celebrate successes. Although much of this work is based in secondary schools the underpinning principles and themes are significant in the primary phase too. These themes include:

- mutual respect;
- strong relationships;

- fairness;
- shared and consistent understanding by all staff and children;
- knowledge of children's needs;
- linking academic and behaviour performance;
- close tracking;
- realistic target setting;
- celebration of success.

Perhaps the most significant theme is that of helping children to reflect on their behaviour and, from this, teaching coping skills to manage the trigger mechanisms that might result in poor behaviour. The philosophy behind this is evident in Blandford's (2000) research, through which she identified the use of a *target book* as a positive strategy. As well as addressing all the themes identified by OFSTED above, this also involves the child in negotiations to agree targets and gives clear messages about how to meet these.

The important role played by parents and carers is emphasised in all literature concerning behaviour management. This role is much more significant than being able to receive a letter outlining their child's misdemeanours, and is more about establishing a reciprocal partnership that extends the community ethos and values to the home. OFSTED (2005b, p19) notes that:

> … where partnerships between parents and schools are strong, parents are involved as soon as concerns arise. Parents are seen as partners rather than being blamed for the poor behaviour of their children.

Interestingly, primary school children also want their parents to be involved both in celebrating achievement and when reprimanded for poor behaviour (Merritt and Tang, 1994). Research into children's views on behaviour management issues also points to the importance of the relationships they have with their teachers. They respond to private comments that are not drawn out or made in such a way as to cause humiliation. This leaves us questioning the effectiveness of common strategies used to manage low-level misbehaviour. It is commonplace in classrooms to have *names on the board*, or other public warning systems. This can only be seen as a form of public humiliation. Research by Houghton, Whedall, Jukes and Sharp (1990) suggests that private rebuke has a positive impact on behaviour. They also suggest that private praise is more effective, and we are left questioning the impact of sticker charts, smiley faces and other forms of public extrinsic motivation.

How?

Before you read the following extract, read:

- Pollard, A (2005) 'How are we managing the class?', in *Readings for reflective teaching*, 2nd edition. London: Continuum.

Extract: Hayes, D (2004) *Foundations of primary teaching, 3rd edition, pp270–72.* London: David Fulton.

Silly behaviour

Very few children are deviant, though some are regular rule-breakers and persistent offenders. Most unacceptable behaviour is due to silliness rather than deviance and takes a number of different forms:

- *Uncontrolled behaviour:* shouting out an answer to a question without permission.
- *Arrogant:* calling out a 'clever' remark.
- *Distractive:* showing off by doing something daring.
- *Detached:* deliberately working very slowly.
- *Spiteful:* teasing another child.
- *Insolent:* asking pointless questions.
- *Deceptive:* pretending not to understand.

These instances are common in some classrooms and are associated with inappropriate work, boredom or general lack of respect. They can signal that it is time to change content, terminate a teaching approach or re-evaluate lesson management. On such occasions it is important that teachers try to understand the behaviour and respond positively. Thus:

Uncontrolled behaviour: children who call out without permission lack self-discipline or do not understand the rules.

Arrogant behaviour: children who call out a silly remark may be signalling a lack of respect for the teacher or simply showing off to impress friends.

Distractive behaviour: children who show off are probably doing so because it is more enjoyable than concentrating on unstimulating work.

Detached behaviour: children who work very slowly may be showing that they are not prepared to engage with uninteresting or unduly demanding activities.

Spiteful behaviour: children who deliberately tease another child are enjoying the power that accompanies ridicule.

Insolent behaviour: children who ask pointless questions are wasting time but avoiding confrontation with the teacher by giving the appearance of interest.

Deceptive behaviour: children who pretend not to understand may be trying to undermine the teacher's authority and create a distraction from the main point of the lesson.

These and similar strategies are used by the small number of children who have decided that messing about is preferable to concentrating on the work; their actions are deliberate but not necessarily serious if attended to appropriately from an early stage. Although teachers rightly feel annoyed by the disruptions, they also act as a warning signal about the need to review the lesson's effectiveness and relevance. It is difficult to make every lesson stimulating and relevant for all children, but persistent boredom not only affects the quality of the children's work but influences their attitudes (Figure 8.1 The consequences of boredom).

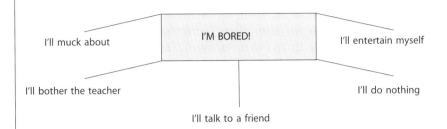

Figure 8.1. The consequences of boredom

Faced with silly behaviour, inexperienced teachers may be tempted to ignore it or hope that by sounding fierce they can minimise the disruption. In fact, ignoring the behaviour is rarely effective (though there are exceptions to this rule, see later) and may indicate to the class that the teacher is not in control of events. Similarly, severe comments often make matters worse in the long term and lead to teacher exhaustion and distress. The problem with harsh reactions is that they deal only with the symptoms and not the underlying causes such as boredom, bravado, inappropriate lessons, inadequate lesson management, and so on. Quite often, these underlying causes take time to diagnose and remedy, so a teacher may have to resort to *holding measures* as a temporary means of counteracting the silly behaviour. Examples of holding methods for each of the above categories of behaviour include the following set of reactions:

Uncontrolled behaviour: 'Olive, you forgot our count to three before you speak rule. Please remember in future.' (The response is merely a statement of fact and avoids attributing blame.)

Arrogant behaviour: 'John. Remember to put your hand up first and take your turn if you've anything to say.' (The response strengthens the teacher's authority, reminds everyone of the rules and avoids confrontation with John.)

Distractive behaviour: 'Please sit still on your chair, Rhoda, we don't want anyone injured thank you.' (The response focuses upon Rhoda's welfare rather than her inappropriate behaviour.)

Detached behaviour: 'Are you finding this difficult, Ellie? Perhaps I can help you along a bit.' (The response allows the teacher to set short-term targets for Ellie.)

Spiteful behaviour: 'If you've got anything to say, Ben, say something kind; otherwise keep quiet. Let's see how helpful you can be for the remainder of the lesson; I'll ask you about it after everyone has gone out.' (The response indicates the teacher's displeasure, sets boundaries upon Ben's behaviour and offers him the chance to redeem himself.)

Insolent behaviour: 'Put your hand up if you think you know the answer to Gordon's question.' (The response focuses upon Gordon's 'ignorance' and allows other children to gain satisfaction from offering the correct answer. An ironic afterthought is also useful: 'It looks as if everybody knew the answer except you, Gordon! You will need to work harder if you want to a keep up with the others.')

Deceptive behaviour: 'If you don't understand by now, Julie, you'd better stay behind after the lesson and I'll explain it to you then.' (The response calls Julie's bluff and puts the onus upon her to complete the work.)

Analysis

This final section moves on to consider some of the practical strategies that teachers can use if they are in a position where they have to deal with poor behaviour. The extract above provides some useful definitions of behaviours and examples of responses, but it should be read in the context of earlier discussions in this chapter and with reference to the in-depth discussions presented in section 11 of Pollard's text, referenced above.

Practical applications and implications

Using Hayes's (2004) definition of *silly behaviour*, think about the children you have observed displaying these types of behaviours. These might be:

- uncontrolled;
- arrogant;
- distractive;
- detached;
- spiteful;
- insolent;
- deceptive.

1. Can you reflect on the reasons why the children might have been behaving in such a manner?

Hayes notes that most of these kinds of behaviour are attributable to the work set, relationships or classroom environment.

2. What strategies would you employ to rectify matters?

While Hayes does go on to provide some practical and professionally appropriate ways of managing on-going silly behaviours, he is also clear that these must be viewed as temporary until a permanent cause and solution can be found. Grossman (2004), writing from a US perspective, maps out a reflective journey that a teacher can take as s/he decides how best to respond to an incident of challenging behaviour. The first decision has to be whether to intervene or not. This will be determined by the motivation behind the behaviour, as it may be unwise or distracting to intervene unnecessarily. According to Grossman, if intervention is required, the action will fall into one of two categories:

1. Immediate intervention, required in response to behaviour that is

- dangerous or harmful;
- destructive;
- likely to deteriorate;
- contagious;
- self-perpetuating.

2. Delayed intervention, when the teacher feels the timing is more appropriate and/or when relevant information has been gathered.

Once an intervention is deemed necessary, the manner in which it is carried out must be considered. It is important to maintain dignity, respect and your relationships with the children. Kyriacou's checklist (1997, p102–103) for dealing with challenging behaviour provides a useful reference point:

- stay calm;
- be aware of the heat of the moment;
- use your social skills;
- design a mutual face saver;
- get help if needed.

While it is important that teachers are able to intervene with immediate effect, it is worth stressing once again that this level of disruptive behaviour is not the norm. The list of strategies referred to in this section should be considered the exception that will be needed very occasionally.

Summary

This chapter concludes this section of the book, and it has explored and dealt with the area that is of greatest concern to new and beginning teachers. There will be occasions where every teacher is required to manage challenging behaviour. The aim of this book is to help in providing a positive learning culture that is grounded in mutual respect where the needs of individual children are known and supported. It is hoped that this ethos and understanding will provide a framework for teachers, so that challenging situations can be seen and managed within a wider context. All too often challenging behaviour is seen as a huge obstacle behind which all other positives are obscured.

The Elton Report (DES, 1989, p8) is a key document in shaping current thinking in this area. In conclusion to this chapter it is important to re-emphasise the inter-linking relationship between school effectiveness (ethos and achievement) and behaviour. Elton states that:

The behaviour of pupils in a school is influenced by every aspect of the way in which it is run and how it relates to the community it serves. It is the combination of all these factors that gives a school its character and identity. Together, they can produce an orderly and successful school in a difficult catchment area; equally, they can produce an unsuccessful school in what should be much easier circumstances.

Further reading

Blandford, S (2005) *Sonia Blandford's masterclass*. London: Sage.

Desforges, C (1995) *An introduction to teaching*. London: Basil Blackwell.

Grossman, H (2004) *Classroom behaviour management for diverse and inclusive schools*, 3rd edition. Oxford: Rowan and Littlefield.

www.behaviour4learning.ac.uk

Section 3: Children and individual needs

9 Spiritual, moral, social and cultural values in the classroom

By the end of this chapter you should have:

- further considered **why** it might be of value to the individual and to society to develop these values and attributes in an education setting;
- reflected on **what** the notions of *spiritual, moral, social* and *cultural* might mean to you as an individual and in what way these interpretations are with you as you teach;
- analysed **how** you might develop your own pedagogy in order to reflect these areas of a child's development.

Linking your learning

- Jacques, K and Hyland, R (2003) *Achieving QTS. Professional studies: primary phase*, Chapter 10. Exeter: Learning Matters.

Professional Standards for QTS
1.7, 2.2, 2.4, 3.3.1, 3.3.6

Introduction

The 1988 *Education Reform Act* (DES, 1988) and the resulting National Curriculum (DES, 1989) placed spiritual, moral, social and cultural (SMSC) development at the core of the aims and purposes of education. The political and social imperatives behind this policy development are still debated and contested nearly 20 years later. This chapter explores those debates in a way that will enable teachers to draw conclusions about their own pedagogy and practice in the classroom.

In order to explore the issues at a meaningful level you will need to be willing to reflect upon your own beliefs and values, and honestly to consider how these are impacting upon your practice as a teacher. It is this process of personal meta-reflection that will foster development for the children you teach and, as a teacher, it is important to act as a positive role model. This is not without difficulty, as each of the areas of SMSC has the potential to raise issues that are personal, sensitive and controversial. Teachers and children need a creative vocabulary with which to communicate their common and unique responses to the *big* questions that everyday life raises. Moments of natural disaster such as the tsunami (2004), or national celebrations such as the triumph of sporting heroes, require schools to be places where children can explore their understanding and questions together in a safe learning environment.

It is also important to appreciate that the terminology, understandings and definitions of SMSC are in themselves contested. Yet it is every teacher's responsibility to make provision for their development in the classroom context. OFSTED's (2003b, p34) inspection framework requires inspectors to judge the extent to which children are enabled to:

- develop self-knowledge and spiritual awareness;
- understand and respect other people's feelings, values and beliefs;
- understand and apply the principles that help distinguish right from wrong;
- understand and fulfil the responsibilities of living in a community;
- appreciate their own and others' cultural traditions.

As you work through this chapter, it will be useful to reflect upon the following two questions:

1. What opportunities have you had in your own education to explore spiritual, moral, social and cultural issues?
2. How far would you feel comfortable about exploring sensitive issues in a classroom context?

Why?

Before you read the following extract, read:

- SCAA (1997) *Findings of the consultation on values in education and the community.* London: HMSO.
- Hay, D and Nye, R (1998) *The spirit of the child.* London: HarperCollins.

These texts provide contrasting viewpoints about the purposes of spiritual development in a school context.

Extract: Bigger, S and Brown, E (1999) *Spiritual, Moral, Social and Cultural Development,* pp4–5. London: David Fulton.

What kind of young people are being turned out by the education system? Youngsters who know facts about academic subjects? Or motivated responsible young adults with a thirst for understanding, a curiosity about life, a concern to contribute to the communities in which they find themselves, and to build relationships with other people? The compulsion to 'reform' education has focused on systems and curriculum, but should not lose sight of how education affects pupils and fits them for the tasks ahead. Which vision of education we choose helps us to create policies and priorities on teaching and learning. There is a tension in British education between many different voices, debating teaching and assessment methods, accountability, relationships between schools and parents, and values.

Schools have been turned upside down by developments stemming from the 1988 Education Reform Act which brought in a National Curriculum of traditional subjects, choosing a vision that pupils should be aware of and interested in these. 'It is quite common for people to excel at subjects yet not have benefited as persons' (Newby 1997, p. 292): this raises the question of the extent to which education should focus on understanding life and the world and our place and role within it – educating the whole person (Erricker *et al.* 1997). As a response, cross-curricular perspectives and themes were put in place, demonstrating how social, personal, environmental, vocational and citizenship perspectives could be introduced. These are of low priority in a crowded school curriculum.

The 1988 Education Reform Act had higher aspirations as is revealed by its opening statement, that the school curriculum should promote the spiritual, moral, cultural, mental and physical development of pupils and to prepare pupils for the opportunities, responsibilities and experiences of adult life. The National Curriculum Council (NCC 1993) produced a discussion paper with a broad secular view of spirituality, and with moral values which 'contain moral absolutes' sounding like a behaviour policy. The Schools Curriculum and Assessment Authority (SCAA) reported on a national conference regarding the place of spiritual and moral development in education for adult life (SCAA 1996). From this came a national forum to advance discussion. The focus on spiritual, moral, social and cultural aspects of education recognises the importance of human experience – of life, of how we think about ourselves, our responsibilities, our place in the world, and our responses to others who are different. Whatever else it does, education should help children understand themselves and their world and enable them to make an informed and responsible contribution to their community and to society. Academic subjects have a part to play, contributing to a school's positive ethos. The Office for Standards in Education (OFSTED) are required to monitor this.

In this book we examine the human side of the school curriculum – both in the formal curriculum which is planned and taught, and the informal curriculum of hidden messages that pupils pick up. If pupils are *taught* justice but experience unfairness in the school system, the informal learning from experience may be the more powerful. The legally prescribed daily act of collective worship can provide a focus for a caring, sharing ethos: but we need a substantial redefinition of 'worship' (usually used in the context of believers) to have an *educational* rather than confessional purpose, for groups of pupils from a range of religious backgrounds or with secular life-stances. A focus on the values discussed here provide a starting point.

Analysis

This extract, along with the suggested preparatory reading above, raises significant questions about the values underpinning education. Values and principles have been raised as an area for consideration in all the chapters of this book, but it is in the spiritual, moral, social and cultural domains that we form, own and live out our values and identity.

Personal response

If you could give your child one gift or quality when s/he leaves school what would it be? (Burns and Lamont, 1995)

Practical implications and activities

1. With a trusted colleague or peer, analyse your personal responses and highlight the similarities and differences.

2. Identify an event reported in the media recently. What values are referred to? What implications might there be for education policy development? How might a school respond to the media reports?

Draw a pen sketch of a school you know well. What are the key values you can identify? Where does your evidence come from: policies or practices?

Bigger and Brown usefully outline the timeline of key events as they relate to education developments and SMSC. Bastide (1999) explores the controversies in more detail and, although he is discussing the development of religious education, many of the issues are related and thus relevant. Key to this discussion is the perception that a religious or spiritual underpinning for education is a means of supporting social cohesion and raising moral standards. Further, there is some sense that *spirituality* replaced the word *religious* in the discourse of education so as to make it more acceptable in a pluralistic and multifaith Britain. Inherently, the majority of theorists and policy makers seem to promote SMSC as a *good thing*.

However, if you then overlay the earlier discussions about the nature of education, the debate becomes more controversial. Is education about the transmission of an accepted body of public knowledge or the construction of meaning and knowledge (see Chapter 8)? If it is about the former, then the power to promote favoured sets of values from a position of authority presents the dangers of indoctrination and exclusion. If, however, it is possible to achieve an open-minded environment where meaning and understanding can be co-constructed, then it provides a rich opportunity to draw on a range of cultural and community views.

What?

Before you read the following extract, read:

- Coles, R (1986) *The moral life of children.* New York: First Atlantic Monthly Press.

This book provides an easily accessible narrative on the moral lives of children – select sections that interest you.

Extract: Erricker, C and Erricker, J (2000) *Reconstructing religious, spiritual and moral education,* **pp89–90. London: RoutledgeFalmer.**

The forum identified a number of values (see box) on which members believed society as a whole would agree. 'Extensive consultation' showed there to be overwhelming agreement on these values. However the nature of that consultation – that is, the actual nature of the questions asked – made it difficult to disagree with the forum's conclusions in that the questions were vague and general. The remit of the forum was to decide whether there are any values that are commonly agreed upon across society, not whether there are any values that should be agreed upon across society. Accordingly the only authority claimed for these values is the authority of consensus.

This remit shows an interesting approach. On the face of it, it conforms with the notion of socially constructed morality, that is, there is no authority claimed for these values except consensus. However, this is not the process of the construction of morality, but an attempt to get people whose moralities have been constructed in different communities to agree that their moralities are the same. Each of these separate moral systems are based on and legitimated by different authorities: the various religious traditions, humanism and so on. The varying philosophies behind the values were ignored and only the discrete, identifiable, common bits were deemed important. There was no suggestion that difference was to be appreciated, lived with and celebrated, but that everything that could not be identified as 'the same' was to be ignored. Thus if we can all agree on a particular value it can be included, but if we do not, however important that value is to our community, it will not be included. The possibility of 'consensus' is obviously remote, and even if it is achieved the value of the agreed values is debatable.

The following quotation shows how the authors of this exercise attempted to address some of the above points:

> These values are not exhaustive. They do not, for example, include religious beliefs, principles or teachings, though these are often the source from which commonly-held values derive. The statement neither implies nor entails that these are the only values that should be taught in schools. There is no suggestion, in particular, that schools should confine themselves to these values.

It is difficult to see which values will remain 'common' after this disclaimer and difficult to see the point of identifying these putative common values. Will the common values be given more emphasis in school? Will they be taught as having more value because they are common? If so, what will be the status of other values that are associated with the traditions?

The next quotation disclaims even more: 'Agreement on the values is also compatible with different interpretations and applications of these values. It is for schools to decide, reflecting the range of views in the wider community, how these values should be interpreted and applied'. Here schools are permitted to interpret and apply the common values as they wish, presumably by putting them back into the context of the traditions and philosophies from whence they came, and from which they were extracted by the processes of the forum. What, therefore, is the point of identifying their commonality?

The document goes on: 'The ordering of these values does not imply any priority or necessary preference. The ordering reflects the belief of many that values in the context of the self must precede the development of other values'. I think this too is problematic. To state that the ordering does not imply priority but 'reflects the belief of many' is to sit on the fence. Either there is no priority, or values in the context of the self are to precede others. The latter statement certainly reflects the standard Kohlbergian theories of moral development.

These values are so fundamental that they may appear unexceptional. Their demanding nature is, however, demonstrated both by our collective failure consistently to live up to them, and the moral challenge that acting on them in practice entails. The values identified by this process of 'consensus' are certainly unexceptional, but this is not because they are fundamental. Our behaviour as a society cannot be said to live up to them, as they are stated here, but this is not because we are moral failures, it is because these values, as stated here, have been reduced by the process of consensus to simplistic, generalised clichés that have no more power or meaning than the stricture 'be good'. Life is so much more complicated than these values give it credit for, and by reducing moral guidance to this level we do our children a great disservice. We run the risk of, once again, having an aspect of education dismissed by pupils because their thinking is at a much more sophisticated level than the curriculum we offer them.

All that this exercise has done is to identify what schools should tell children to do. It does not offer any help in the difficult task of justifying this prescription to the children, explaining why they should hold the values that have been identified or help in developing the emotional skills that the children will need in order to live by these values.

The Errickers are firm and outspoken in their criticism of the consultation process that was undertaken to arrive at the set of statements that schools are encouraged to address in order to promulgate the 'agreed' values. These have been interpreted for the inspectorate to try to promote some sense of common understanding and equity in the inspection process. For the purposes of this book they provide an interesting focus for these discussions.

Spiritual development is the development of the non-material element of a human being which animates and sustains us and, depending on our point of view, either ends or continues in some form when we die. It is about the development of a sense of identity, self-worth, personal insight, meaning and purpose. It is about the development of a pupil's 'spirit'. Some people may call it the development of a pupil's 'soul', others the development of 'personality' or 'character' (OFSTED, 2004, p12).

Moral development is about the building, by pupils, of a framework of moral values that regulates their personal behaviour. It is also about the development of pupils' understanding of society's shared and agreed values. It is about understanding that there are issues where there is disagreement and it is also about understanding that society's values change. Moral development is about gaining an understanding of the range of views and the reasons for the range. It is also about developing an opinion about different views (OFSTED, 2004, p15).

It is clear that the Errickers, who adopt a social constructivist approach to learning, do not see sufficient space for children to negotiate and make meaning if they are to work to definitions such as those above. The focus in teachers' minds ought to be upon equipping the children with the skills to be able to reflect, interpret and communicate their own views with a developed emotional strength.

The work of the Errickers has been widely criticised by pragmatists and those searching to include a faith-based interpretation of matters moral and spiritual. Thatcher (1999) and Wright (2000) find, for differing reasons, that a child-centred spirituality that rejects a fixed faith-based perspective is not one that can be supported. However, it seems appealing to encompass spiritual and moral, as well as cultural and social, development within an open and creating community, where the teachers and children are empowered to create a shared identity, and are prepared and supported to take risks.

How?

Before you read the following extract, read:

- Lewisham Education Service (1999) *SMSC – providing for spiritual, moral, social and cultural development of pupils.* London: Lewisham Education Service.
- Inman, S, Buck, M and Burke, H (1998) *Assessing personal and social development: measuring the unmeasurable.* London: RoutldegeFalmer.

Both of these texts provide discussions and practical applications for some of the issues discussed in the following section.

Extract: Grainger, T and Kendall-Seatter, S (2003) 'Drama and spirituality: reflective connections', *International Journal of Children's Spirituality,* **8 (1), pp26–29.**

Exploring the potential of drama in spiritual development

In classroom drama, children search for meaning and purpose in fictional settings and learn more about the real world from their improvisational engagement in an imaginary one. Drama involves making and shaping new worlds and investigating issues within them, so it has considerable potential as a tool in the development of spirituality. The opportunity for 'innerstanding' (Heathcote and Bolton, 1995) and inhabiting the lives of others, enables children to experience safe emotional engagement and take part in creative explorations of secular and faith tales. In classroom drama, children create and experience a living narrative and examine it from within. Their teacher, often in role, accompanies the learners on this journey and uses a range of conventions to investigate the themes, characters, motives and meanings in the text. Such investigations can also support the creation of community, the development of self-knowledge and may involve opportunities to engage in feelings of wonder and transcendence. Teaching and learning are more holistically encountered in the context of drama and elements of drama are recognisable in Bowness and Carter's (1999) description of the process of spiritual learning. They suggest there should be an

emphasis on intuition, experience, imagination, silence in the face of mystery, wondering, open exploration, being as well as doing, reflecting, giving 'space for the spirit', holism and making connections. (p. 226)

Improvisational classroom drama can encompass all of these features as it acknowledges that teaching and learning are not merely cognitive but emotional, aesthetic and ethical acts. To explore the opportunities which drama offers spiritual development, a vignette from the classroom is recounted and interpreted. It was undertaken with Year 5 children, aged 9 and 10 and was based upon the persecution of the Israelites in Egypt, as recounted in the Bible, Exodus 1 and 2. As the drama unfolds, the learning is analysed and exemplified in relation to aspects of spirituality. These include meaning and purpose, transcendence, self-knowledge and relationships (NCC, 1993). In addition to the work of others, the 'framework for children's spirituality' (Hay and Nye, 1998) formed an important reference point for the analysis. In order to hear the voices of the children and appreciate the power of the drama, the analysis and reflection is quite deliberately presented separately, it generally follows each section of the dramatic action.

In essence, the tale tells of how the Egyptian Pharaoh at that time developed a sense of insecurity, amounting to paranoia over the number of Israelites in his land. Concerned lest they should join his enemies or plot against him, he made them work as slaves. The people of Israel flourished, however, so he ordered that the Hebrew midwives should kill all newborn males. The midwives, not wishing to become child murderers, tricked the Pharaoh and finally his soldiers were commanded to act. The story tells of how Jochebed and Amram, an Israelite couple, placed their son in a cradle of rushes and trusted God to look after him. Although this class had undoubtedly heard the tale of Moses before, this drama session sought to explore the social and moral issues in the narrative, as well as expand the children's knowledge and understanding of persecution. Classroom drama does not require the learner to re-enact the known, but involves discovering the unknown and exploring situations, values, motives, thoughts and feelings. Although the session was not planned with the conscious aim of facilitating spiritual development, when the drama was examined the seemingly elusive nature of spirituality and the children's learning in this domain became more evident. It is clear that improvisational drama may hold a valuable key to unlocking a range of processes, strategies and consequences for enriching children's spiritual development.

'It's our land, our harvest, we should share it': spirituality as community

Initially, the teacher sought to build a sense of community both fictionally and for real through the drama, which as Taggart (2001) intimates, must be a core practice for all of us who desire spirituality in education. Hull (1995) insists that 'spirituality seeks to recreate community through participation in the lives of others' (p. 132). In creating the drama context, the teacher helped the class build a sense of the place and the people involved. They discussed the kinds of jobs folk in the Egyptian farming community would do, mimed these, then worked in groups creating contrasting freeze frames to show farmers in times of plenty and of hardship. The teacher took on the role of an Egyptian foreman arriving in the fields to demand the 'first fruits' of the harvest as payment to the Pharaoh for the use of his land. As family groups, the learners gathered together to decide what they would offer the Pharaoh. Immediately some began to grumble and complain, whispering amongst themselves about ways to avoid this tax or withhold their resources. An empty chair was used symbolically for children to give witness to the rest of the class about their motives, behaviour and attitudes at this time. Several voiced the view that the Pharaoh could not be trusted, and argued that once the pattern was established he would demand more; others felt the land belonged to all the people and its harvest should be shared. Connections were then made to contemporary life, allowing a pause outside the imaginary frame. This reflective discussion was quite lengthy, and included the existence and fairness of council taxes, as well as giving up personal material possessions, e.g. Gameboys and Nintendos, photos of loved ones and so on. As Nathan perceptively observed, 'You could give away your photos 'cos they'll still be with you in your heart, won't they?' The children's engagement and reflection in the drama had prompted imaginative connections to emerge in the form of text to life and life to text moves (Meek, 1988) and allowed the meanings they constructed to be both relevant and real. Within this empathetically created reality, the children were apparently demonstrating many of the implicit strategies (reasoning, imagining, moralising) that researchers such as Hay and Nye (1998) argue are vital for a maturing spirituality.

'What have we ever done to them?': explaining meaning and purpose

Many of the group depictions showed the Israelites in hiding. Notes and quick diary entries were written which reflected the thoughts and fears of those awaiting the possible arrival of the soldiers. These reveal the affective involvement of the children, since although the world of drama is fictional, the children's responses and feelings became increasingly real as the pressure of the dramatic moment brought their feelings to the fore. It is clear too that the children used this writing to make sense of the situation in which they found themselves.

> "I don't know what is happening. My mum just told us to hide, my heart is beating so loudly surely they will hear."

> "I hear footsteps outside, who do they want? Just the boys? What have we ever done to them? I wish we had left when we had the chance."

The questioning stance reflected in these two examples shows how the meanings developed in the drama had begun to be considered. Improvised drama is a particularly rich medium for exploring multiple meanings and the gaps in the text which leave room for ambiguity and do not effect closure. (Iser, 1978)

> "I cannot tell you where we are. But I have taken Thoremu to the best hiding place there is. Thoremu thinks it's just a game. I told him it is and we have to be quiet or else they will find us."

> "The soldiers are getting closer every minute. It's dark. I hear houses being ripped apart and babies screaming. I can't help myself. I start to cry."

The power in the latter examples lies both in their reflective tenor and their emotionally positioned stance within the drama. Through sharing their writing and their views about the situation in reflective time outside the frame of the drama, it was clear that their strong feelings and imaginative involvement seemed to have fuelled the processes of identification and transformation. In discussing the perspectives of the terrified Israelites and connecting to the 'special fear' of hide and seek, scenes on the news and moments when parents had made them afraid, the children were co-authoring this text from the inside, making sense and constructing meaning together.

Grainger and Kendall-Seatter go on to analyse further themes evident in this case-study example of a classroom exploration of spirituality through drama and story. The real engagement of the learners is evident, and they are genuinely involved in creating their own interpretations and responses. The medium of drama is ideal in that it naturally provides open learning opportunities where the answer is not known in advance or prescribed.

A recurring theme in this book is the role and voice of the learner. Sections 1 and 2 suggested that the learner's input should be evident in curriculum planning and assessment, the creation of the classroom ethos and the associated routines and rituals. This case study illustrates the same potential as the children explore:

- spirituality as community;
- self-knowledge through relationships;
- explanations of meaning and purpose;
- the experience of feelings of transcendence.

The opportunity to create a fictional world, enter it and then explore the issues and dilemmas from within provides a good example of a secure learning environment in which children are safe to take risks.

Working in such a way is not without challenge for the teacher. The ability to go into role with a group of children will be reliant on a trusting and respectful relationship, high motivation levels and resulting low levels of disruptive behaviour. It is important that such activities are planned carefully even though the temptation may be to leave them unplanned to retain flexibility. The confidence to engage in these activities comes from the teacher, who can work with the class to explore opportunities that they have anticipated, but not lead them to a point that he or she has pre-planned.

The advisory material from Lewisham LEA is a good example of supporting materials that point to the potential for SMSC across the curriculum.

Practical implications and activities

The following list was compiled by teachers reflecting upon teaching styles and SMSC in their schools:

- build good relationships with pupils;
- value each individual;
- use open questions;
- encourage independent learning;
- be prepared to be child-like to share the joys felt by the children;
- use role play;
- teachers need to be seen to be learners.
  (Adapted from Brown and Seaman, 2001)

---

1. Which of these have you tried in the classroom? What happened?

2. As you develop your own pedagogy for SMSC, where do your strengths and areas for development lie when you consider your teaching style?

3. Using a mapping grid, brainstorm opportunities for SMSC across the curriculum.

4. What opportunities does this suggest for:

    - cross-curricular working?
    - the development of skills, attitudes and processes?
    - planning for continuity and progression?

Summary

This chapter has challenged you to explore your own values and beliefs and how these will influence the way you come to your work in the classroom. SMSC is perhaps one of the most debated and contested areas in contemporary educational discourse. Moves to introduce citizenship and personal, social and health education (PSHE) (QCA, 1998a), via non-statutory frameworks that sit alongside the National Curriculum (DfEE/QCA, 1999) have caused the debate around SMSC to surface again. It could be argued that, with such a consensus view of SMSC filtering through to school practice and resulting in detachment from any explicit religious or cultural identity (Erricker and Erricker, 2000), what remains is good citizenship education. This controversial viewpoint does not support the development of a child's sense of identity or attachment to any community or cultural heritage that has a faith dimension. Above all, it is of paramount importance that SMSC is viewed, not as a bank of knowledge content, but as a participation-led element of the primary curriculum. As this list adapted from the work of Brown and Furlong (1996) indicates, facilitating spiritual development is active, and involves the children in:

- recognising the existence of others;
- becoming aware;
- reflecting on experience;
- questioning and exploring meanings;
- understanding and evaluating a range of responses;
- developing personal views;
- applying insights gained.

Further reading

Best, R (ed) (1996) *Education, spirituality and the whole child.* London: Continuum.

Brown, A and Seaman, A (2001) *Feeding minds and touching hearts: Spiritual development in the primary school.* London: RMEP.

Burns, S and Lamont, G (1997) *Values and visions.* London: Hodder and Stoughton.

Erricker, C, Erricker, J, Ota, C, Sullivan, D and Fletcher, M (1997) *The Education of the whole child.* London: Cassell.

10 Equal opportunities in the school

By the end of this chapter you should have:

- further considered **why** it is important that teachers acknowledge and reflect on their own views and prejudices in an education setting;
- reflected on **what** issues and debates come to bear when considering evidence around achievement and equal opportunities;
- analysed **how** you might develop your own pedagogy in a way that is grounded in reflective practice that constantly challenges prejudice.

Linking your learning

- Jacques, K and Hyland, R (2003) *Achieving QTS. Professional studies: primary phase*, Chapter 11. Exeter: Learning Matters.

Professional Standards for QTS
1.1, 1.2, 1.8, 3.3.14

Introduction

Hyland's chapter in Jacques and Hyland (2003) provides a good overview of definitions and of the relevant legislative reference points relating to equal opportunities issues in school. The focus of this chapter is on supporting teachers to reflect on their own views and how to address them in their teaching. The example of good practice in this chapter relates to gender issues, but the generic themes are transferable to other categories including:

- race;
- colour;
- nationality;
- ethnic origin;
- religion;
- disability;
- sexual orientation.

As has been noted in Sections 1 and 2, schools reflect the community in which they are situated and, for learning to be effective, they need to respond and contribute to that community. In doing so they will develop their own ethos which is a rich and unique blend of the people in the school. This is captured by Maden (2002, p308), who reflects that:

> ... schools represent, transmit and sometimes challenge a dense and complex conflation of social and educational history, as well as current expectations and norms. Schools are where society's hopes and fears are concentrated and synthesised into a daily set of transactions involving all our children.

As you read this chapter, reflect on the underlying themes by exploring the questions below.

1. What is the role of the child's voice when that might express controversial prejudices?

2. What are my own prejudices and where might these have come from?

Why?

Before you read the following extract, read.

- Pollard, A, (ed) (2002) *Readings for reflective teaching*, Section 15. London: Continuum.

This section of material provides a set of readings that challenge you to explore key issues around equal opportunities.

Extract: Gaine, C (1995) *Still no problem here*, pp11–12. Stoke-on-Trent: Trentham Books

Before the reader goes off to try and get responses like those I have reported here for her- or himself I would like to issue a warning: even if similar views are revealed, many colleagues in the same school, teaching the same children, simply will not believe that significant levels of hostility exist. Their resistance seems to me to be for one or a combination five reasons.

First, colleagues may not have examined their own assumptions and conceptions about 'race', immigration, and prejudice, so the things pupils say might not grate on their ears the way they would on others'. For those who do not consider this issue important, pupils' attitudes are simply part of the background noise; they do not register.

Second, teachers are generally aware that this can be an explosive issue and not easy to handle in a classroom, or fear that doing so 'will make things worse.' An HMI document based on meetings held in five LEAs found that

> … there was general agreement that race relations in schools were a matter of considerable concern, and that there was a need to respond to this concern (1983:p.3).

It also found that teachers may ignore things because 'racism is difficult and sensitive territory', and Swann often found the same. There has been considerable development work in many largely-white LEAs over the past decade, many whole school initiatives on 'race' in particular or equal opportunities in general, more interest in initial teacher education and a reasonable range of stimulus and support materials from publishing and TV, yet the fact remains that it is difficult, it does cause anxiety in teachers, and it this produces a powerful temptation to leave well alone.

Third, some will argue (with politicians', media, LEA, governors', heads' and parental support in many cases) that it is no business of the school to go into controversial matters of this sort. There is certainly plenty of ebb and flow in the 'official' support this issue receives. The Education Reform Act's preamble seems to say that such social concerns are the business of education; the later compilation of the actual curriculum tacitly said it was not. John Major said (with reference to Cheltenham's black candidate in the 1993 election) that racism had no place in the Tory party but, at the 1992 party conference, he said that student teachers should not spend time studying the politics of class, race and gender. Perhaps some of those most anxious about opening this particular Pandora's Box would rather it was not there at all, so they deny its existence or its rightful place in school.

Fourth, teachers are usually telling the truth when they say they have never heard children expressing racist attitudes. Particularly in white schools it does not tend to arise as a public issue in chemistry, or typing, or when doing minibeasts. I always used to be struck by reactions to Grange Hill, not its 'race' content specifically but the fact that pupils seemed to like it while teachers seldom saw it as anything but an annoying travesty of school life. So it is, from the teachers' point of view, but for large numbers of children school is the backdrop against which they act out the important things in their lives: friendships, crises, group values, conflicts. The important things happen between lessons, in Grange Hill and in real schools, and we teachers are seldom privy to this world.

Fifth, teachers in white areas often point to the small numbers of Asian or black children in the school as indications that there is 'no problem'. 'Jasvir is very well integrated,' 'Carol was elected class representative,' 'Balvinder's best friend is a white girl' and so on. In fact this is entirely beside the point. Children (and adults) are easily capable of having positive feelings about individuals they know, but simultaneously holding generalised negative attitudes about the group that person belongs to. Individual black or Asian children are frequently told, 'Oh you're alright, it's all the others. . .'

All these reasons are important factors in people's resistance to the idea that 'race' has much to do with education for whites — for the ethnic majority. Teachers' anxiety about controversy, their often genuine unawareness of pupils' attitudes, the apparent 'integration' of the few black and Asian pupils, can all collude with our own unexamined prejudices to produce a pernicious conspiracy of inaction.

Analysis

The book from which this is taken gives shocking and illuminating voice to those who have witnessed and experienced racism in schools that do not reflect a multicultural community. Gaine insists that children are being *dangerously misinformed* (p10). He is adamant that teachers do not take these issues seriously and lists a range of reasons, some of which are out of the teacher's direct control.

Gaine argues that teachers are not required to explore their own prejudices and lack of knowledge and thus are, perhaps, unaware of the issues that present themselves in school. Interestingly, this book was written prior to the latest version of the training curriculum for teachers. The government standards state explicitly that Newly Qualified Teachers (NQTs) must be able to:

recognise and respond effectively to equal opportunities issues as they arise in the classroom, including challenging stereotyped views, and by challenging bullying or harassment. (TTA, 2003c, 3.3.14)

This sets the agenda for teacher training curricula, which are audited through the OFSTED inspection process (OFSTED, 2003b). Thus the requirement and quality assurance mechanisms are in place to ensure equal opportunities training is provided for new teachers. However, much training is located in the school context – some employment-based routes are exclusively so – and one might question the extent to which the *no problem here* mantra (Gaine, 1995) might still exist in practice.

Gaine's analysis of teachers' reactions also refers to a desire to *leave well alone* when it comes to racial issues (p11). I would suggest that this might allude to a bigger issue. Our previous chapter explored a similar reaction to matters spiritual and moral. Since the introduction of the National Curriculum (1988), and the subsequent strategies for literacy and numeracy (1998), schools have been legally required to focus on the cognitive aspects of the curriculum – the results of which have been publicised in league tables and inspection reports. Perhaps this has provided an *excuse* to avoid the sensitive and emotive elements of school policy and practice. However, with a renewed interest in learning styles and the emphasis on the affective in education, schools cannot afford to ignore equal opportunities issues. Children learn more effectively when they feel safe and included.

Personal response

Reflect on a school you have worked in.

- Can you recall an incident or occurrence that raised concerns about equal opportunities provision?
- What was the response of the children, staff and others involved?
- Did the school have an equal opportunities policy? Was it evident in practice?

What?

Before you read the following extract, read:

- English, E and Newton, L (2005) *Professional studies in the primary school*, Chapter 9. London: David Fulton.

This chapter provides a useful overview of equal opportunities within the context of the needs of the individual.

Extract: Blair, M (2002) 'Education for all', in Cole, M (ed) (2002) *Professional Values and Practice for Teachers and Student Teachers*, 2nd edition, pp10–13. London: David Fulton.

It would probably be unusual to find a teacher who was not committed to raising the achievement of his or her pupils. Why then would such a condition exist in the

Standards for qualified teacher status? The probable reason lies, once again, in the racial and ethnic dimensions of academic achievement. Reviews of research by Gillborn and Gipps (1996) and Gillborn and Mirza (2000) have shown the persistence of underachievement among some minority ethnic groups over the years. There is no single explanation for this. Writers have variously pointed to issues of language acquisition, to social class, gender, racism and to an interplay of all these, as significant factors in pupil achievement. An important point made by many social analysts and educators is that teaching is a middle-class profession perpetuating middle-class values and therefore excluding in its processes and underlying assumptions, pupils from working-class backgrounds (Sharp and Green 1984). Furthermore, in a society where the bulk of the teaching profession is white, then the interaction of 'race' and class mediates in a powerful way the relationships between minority ethnic group pupils and their teachers (Sleeter 1995).

The exhortation that teachers be committed to the achievement of their pupils is rooted in an implicit acknowledgement of the role of stereotypes,in influencing teachers' beliefs, attitudes and actions. Research shows that such stereotypes affect teachers' relationships with very young children. Connolly (1995), for example, detailed the ways in which six-year-old boys of Caribbean background were labelled and the effects of this labelling on teachers' attitudes towards them. Stereotypes of black men prevalent in the wider society were just as likely to be used against these boys so that they were constructed not only as sexually deviant, but as behaviour problems needing and deserving more stringent control than their white and/or Asian peers.

Individual teachers and schools use many strategies for raising achievement generally and some have developed imaginative and innovative ways to engage their pupils from different social and ethnic backgrounds. Researchers have found that an important method for motivating and encouraging students is to investigate the social and cultural interests of pupils and to incorporate these into one's teaching. Teachers use folk tales, histories, pop and football stars, hip hop music and whatever is topical among pupils or in their communities to bring relevance to points they wish to illustrate in their teaching of various subjects (OFSTED 2002; Blair and Bourne 1998; Ladson-Billings 1995). Important too is the need to understand the barriers to learning for one's pupils. For example, having an afternoon homework club or revision class may be an important strategy. However, unless one monitors take-up of such provision, there is no guarantee that those who need such provision make the most of such opportunities. Boys will often not take advantage of these resources for fear of being labelled swots, or nerds. The teacher or school needs to engage with these fears and find ways of encouraging boys to take up such opportunities. Where particular pupils never seem to take advantage of extra resources provided by the school, it is worth investigating the personal circumstances of the pupil to see whether there are factors in the home or in the school which might be creating difficulties for the pupil. Where a pupil's homework is consistently poor, is it possible they do not have facilities at home for homework? This can be a real issue for refugees or asylum seekers who might live in inadequate temporary homes where a simple item such as a table is a luxury (Virani 2002).

There could be many other factors. For example, is it possible that the pupil is being bullied? Are pupils of Gypsy/Traveller background afraid to come to afterschool activities for fear of harassment? Do some pupils live too far from the school to take advantage of what is on offer? Do such opportunities clash with other community or religious activities such as visits to the Mosque? Commitment to raising achievement is therefore about going one step further in one's efforts to make sure that all pupils are given an equal chance to succeed. Providing equality of opportunity is not only about neutral provision of access but ensuring that the outcomes are also fair.

It is becoming increasingly accepted that in order to have a clear picture of whether differential achievement occurs along ethnic, class, gender, disability or other lines, monitoring by ethnicity, class etc. is important. In addition therefore to tracking individual performance, such monitoring provides a picture of group factors and allows the school to see what other value-added factors affect pupils. The Pupil Level Annual School Census (PLASC) through which schools collect and update information on their pupils is a useful tool for cross-checking different kinds of information about a pupil. For example, one is able to take attendance information about pupils from different groups and examine it against gender, SEN and free school meals (as an indicator of social class) in order to provide a more refined picture of truancy in the school.

Free school meals are, however, a crude measure of social class especially as some pupils (especially in Secondary school) who qualify may not take up this service for fear of being ridiculed. It might be necessary therefore, to take, for example exclusion information of Caribbean heritage boys, and set that against free school meals but also against knowledge of the pupil's family circumstances (single parent, poverty, housing, street code or address) in order to get a better understanding of which black boys are most affected by exclusion. A similar exercise can be carried out in relation to information about other groups such as truancy levels among white boys.

Conclusion

Technical competencies in teaching are important but not sufficient in a diverse, class-based, gendered, multi-ethnic, multi-faith, multilingual society. Teachers now need to think in more complex multi-dimensional ways in order to promote a culture of inclusiveness in the classroom and in the school as a whole. This is necessary if one is to fulfil the requirements of QTS set out above. A 'colour blind' approach, that is, an approach that assumes that all pupils are the same and require the same treatment or provision, overlooks the needs and learning requirements of many pupils. On the other hand, an approach which overemphasises differences between pupils, is in danger of creating fixed ethnic or other enclaves which construct groups as 'other' and in the process, marginalises or excludes them. How is the teacher to achieve the balance of perspective that promotes social justice and fairness for all pupils?

Analysis

Blair (2002) reports that children (especially black children) do not feel respected by their teachers. While this may not be intentional, it is vital that teachers understand the importance of being a role model for their children, even if they themselves are not always shown respect by children. Blair provides some strategies that might support teachers to make explicit their respect for the children. Helpfully, Blair's views and advice are grounded in the principle that respectful behaviour will flow from a commitment to raising standards for all children.

A central theme in Blair's extract is the impact of teachers' stereotyping attitudes upon children's performance and, while it may make uncomfortable reading, the issue is significant. Pollard (2005) challenges teachers not to rest on common sense to inform their practice. Instead he encourages teachers to engage in reflective practice. This is identifiable by seven characteristics in teaching.

1. An active concern with aims and consequences.
2. A cyclical or spiralling process, in which teachers monitor, evaluate and revise their own practice continuously.
3. Evidence-based classroom enquiry.
4. Attitudes of open-mindedness, responsibility and wholeheartedness.
5. Teacher judgement based on evidence-based enquiry and insights from other research.
6. Collaboration and dialogue with colleagues.
7. Creative mediation of externally developed frameworks.
    (p14)

If we overlay Blair's call to explore our own beliefs and prejudices with Pollard's reflective cycle, we should have a powerful tool to confront the stereotypes in our classrooms and, in so doing, raise the achievement and aspirations of the children we are teaching. This is a resource-intensive process, and it may be appropriate for schools to invest in mentoring and peer-coaching forms of professional development to create a culture where teachers are able, as part of their normal routine, to have conversations with colleagues about their developing practice in relation to equal opportunities.

Practical activities and implications

1. Use the following list to reflect on the equal opportunities 'categories':

    - race;
    - colour;
    - nationality;
    - ethnic origin;
    - religion;
    - disability;
    - sexual orientation.

2. Rate your awareness and confidence as a teacher.

3. Go back to a scheme of work you have developed and taught. How could you rework it to support and develop equal opportunities issues through the curriculum?

How?

Before you read the following extract, read:

- **www.multiverse.ac.uk**

This website is an active and growing bank of resources that explore diversity issues in relation to education.

Extract: DfES (2003) *Using the National Healthy School Standard to Raise Boys' Achievement*. pp11-13

www.standards.dfes.gov.uk/genderandachievement/

nhss_boys_achievement2.pdf?version=1)

3. Curriculum planning and resourcing

The broad and balanced curriculum and the requirements of programmes of study need to be sympathetic to both genders. *A school can be said to be working towards raising boys' achievement when, for example*:

- **Schemes of work are developed identifying pupils' learning outcomes** – *and specifically if* – each lesson begins with a clear statement of intended learning outcomes (as exemplified in the Numeracy, Literacy and Key Stage 3 Strategies). For example, in order for many boys to commit themselves to doing a particular piece of work with any real purpose, they need to be totally clear about what is expected and why.

- **An appropriate range of resources is used (including National Grid for Learning sites such as Wired for Health** (www.wiredforhealth.gov.uk), **children's literature and the school nursing service)** – *and specifically if* – all subject areas/coordinators and pastoral staff are responsible for analysing resources for gender and cultural bias. Pupils are also involved in this process, which helps them understand the kind of young people the school is trying to nurture, producing a double benefit. This might profitably be carried out during lesson time.

- **A code of practice for working with external agencies is developed and its implementation monitored** – *and specifically when* – school clearly recognises that, in relation to boys, sound male role models who value learning are particularly useful. The school needs to show that it is obviously aware of gender implications and the messages, both subliminal and overt, when welcoming groups of outsiders into the school.

Further examples of good practice in this area can be found in the Appendix (page 27).

4. Teaching and learning

Good quality teaching is crucial for all pupils. However, every individual has preferred ways of working and styles of learning. Three commonly understood ways of learning are visual, auditory and kinaesthetic. These terms describe the ways in which pupils engage with and make sense of experiences, ie by hearing, seeing or doing.

Research shows that there are generally significant differences between the ways in which most boys and girls prefer to learn. The fact that many schools tend to underplay kinaesthetic learning can be particularly significant for many boys. Schools need to move towards a fuller understanding of pupils' preferred teaching and learning styles. Classroom-based research, surveys or interviews, and discussions in class or at school council could be helpful in this process. *A school can be said to be working towards raising boys' achievement when, for example*:

- **A range of teaching styles** in all lessons **is used such as circle time and debating forums, appropriate to pupils' age, ability and level of maturity** – *and specifically* – if boys are being given the opportunity to be more responsive and achieve more because:

    - Work is delivered in bite-sized chunks and is time-limited
    - Lessons are broken down into a number of different activities, including more active learning opportunities, eg drama, investigation, research or the use of information communication technology (ICT)
    - The work feels relevant to them, with a *real* purpose and a *real* audience
    - Work is delivered with pace and there is a real sense of direction and progression
    - There is an element of challenge or competition, with short-term goals
    - Social learning is allowed from simply sitting with someone who can help them discuss and reflect on ideas, to well organised and structured group work
    - A period of reflection/review is allowed at the end of lessons such as literacy and mathematics lesson plenary sessions
    - Positive feedback is given regularly
    - Cross-curricular literacy initiatives (as recommended by the National Literacy and Key Stage 3 Strategies) encourage more speaking and listening activities, modelling of written tasks, writing frames/'scaffolding'.

- **Recognition is given to different styles of learning and opportunities are offered to put learning into practice such as practical experience in the community and in work** – *for example where* – boys are required to pass on newly learnt skills, eg explaining ICT processes to younger pupils or displaying an end product incorporating an element of self-assessment and review.

- **Peer support for learning is encouraged such as older pupils working with younger ones** – *for example where* – Shared Reading or Buddy Reading is gainfully employed, where older boys with low self-esteem but some reading ability help younger boys with less ability (other schemes, such as Reading Champions and Reading the Game, are also described at www.literacytrust.org.uk).

- **The importance of a safe and supportive teaching environment is recognised where pupils and teachers can work together to promote healthy learning, for example, working agreements are established and classroom layout is considered** – *for example where* – ground rules are established in the classroom for learning as well as behaviour. For example, whole school seating policies that address the arrangement of pupils in any lesson for the purpose of improving learning. It is made clear that seating arrangements can always be reviewed.

- **Pupils are encouraged to consider levels of risk and make informed judgements about their actions** – *for example where* – boys (who tend to be the greatest risk-takers in class) are encouraged to take more considered risks in question-and-answer sessions, through being allowed a few minutes to discuss their answer with a partner before responding.

Analysis

This extract is taken from a comprehensive package of support for teachers. The aim is to provide guidance on how to *address the current gender gap in pupil performance and is intended to support self-review* (DfES, 2003d, p4). This documentation is useful for teachers and is also illustrative of the way forward for education. It demonstrates the link between education and health provision, both in terms of how health impacts upon performance and also in the way that the *Every Child Matters* (2003) legislation will see inter-agency and inter-professional working as commonplace and statutory.

While the extract focuses on the curriculum and learning and teaching strategies, the emphasis is very much upon a whole-school approach, where there is shared ownership and understanding of the values and ethos operating in the school.

Practical activities and implications

The following strategies are identified (DfES, 2003d) as supporting boys' achievement:

- active learning including use of drama, investigation, research, ICT;
- lessons that are broken down into short, well-paced sections with clear aims and purpose;
- content that is relevant to the interests of the pupils;
- positive feedback and time for reflection are included.

Select a single lesson plan that you have developed. Can you rework it, keeping the learning intentions the same, but with reference to the points above?

Smith (2004) explores the debate around boys' underachievement in more depth. Interestingly, she suggests that, traditionally, boys' failings have been attributed to external factors whereas girls' failings have been related to internal factors. Girls' success has been put down to the teacher or context. Smith goes on to state that:

> the received wisdom is that most girls succeed at school because they are compliant and some boys underachieve because they are alienated. (p172)

She suggests that this alienation is close to the risk-taking required to develop higher-order thinking skills. With this in mind, it is worth reviewing the strategies advocated above. The content, pace and structuring of lessons need careful consideration to ensure that teachers balance the need for a safe and secure learning environment with the need for children to take risks. It would appear that this is vital in order for boys to achieve their full potential.

Summary

This chapter has explored a range of issues around equal opportunities, but a theme that has emerged is the importance of teachers confronting, challenging and reflecting upon their own beliefs and prejudices. There is a need for this to be an ongoing, explicit and collaborative reflection that is open-minded and able to influence change. The government is placing an increasing emphasis upon equal opportunities in all sectors of education. Its interest is manifest in guidance documentation such as that produced by the Department of Health (2003), and also in legislative and inspection frameworks. However, there are some important reminders:

- behaviours are not predetermined, but socially constructed;
- each child needs to develop his or her own sense of identity;
- generalisations about behaviour and achievement are not helpful;
- teachers' own attitudes and beliefs influence the way they respond;
- children in school need role models that reflect diversity;
- reflective talk is a key tool.
  (adapted from Smith, 2004, p179)

Further reading

Browne, A and Haylock, D (eds) (2004) *Professional issues for primary teachers.* London: Paul Chapman Publishing.

Epstein, D, Elwood, J, Hey, V and Maw, J (eds) (1999) *Failing boys? Issues in gender and achievement.* Buckingham: OUP.

Gaine, C and George, R (1999) *Gender, 'race' and class in schooling: A new introduction.* London: Falmer.

11 Special educational needs and the teacher

By the end of this chapter you should have:

- further considered **why** it is important that teachers acknowledge and reflect on their own prejudices and fears in relation to special educational needs (SEN);
- reflected on **what** historical and social debates influence current policy and practice;
- analysed **how** you might develop your own pedagogy in a way that is grounded in reflective practice that constantly challenges prejudice.

Linking your learning

- Jacques, K and Hyland, R (2003) *Achieving QTS. Professional studies: primary phase*, Chapter 12. Exeter: Learning Matters.

Professional Standards for QTS

2.6, 3.2.4, 3.3.4

Introduction

Horsfall's chapter in Jacques and Hyland provides a two-part introduction to special educational needs (SEN). As well as introducing the key *categories* of SEN in the mainstream class, he discusses the legislative framework, and how teachers need to work to ensure they are providing an effective learning experience for all children in their care. This chapter aims to take your understanding of SEN forward by encouraging you to engage in some of the issues and debates surrounding this contentious area of education provision. For a more detailed discussion of SEN, please refer to Soan's (2005) parallel title *Achieving QTS. Reflective reader: Primary special educational needs*.

One of my roles is to conduct interview talks for intending primary school teachers, and I can guarantee that I am always asked a question about whether students can specialise in SEN as part of their training. SEN is also a focal point in post-observation tutorials with students on school placement. It seems, among new teachers, that there is a keen interest and desire to want to understand and learn about children with SEN. This may be stimulated by a fear of children who are different and an ignorance of how best to support them in school (Garner and Davies, 2001). Alternatively, it may be driven by a sense of vocation – to want to support those for whom learning may present more challenges.

This chapter continues to develop the theme of meta-reflection, by asking teachers to confront their own views and prejudices, share with colleagues and move their practice forward in a collaborative and honest manner. As you read through it, it will be useful to reflect on two underpinning themes:

1. Where do I stand in relation to inclusion in mainstream schools?

2. What are my own prejudices and where might these have come from?

Why?

Before you read the following extract, read:

- Hume, T (2005) 'Different needs and different responses', in English, E and Newton, L (eds) *Professional studies in the primary school.* London: David Fulton.

This chapter provides key definitions and strategies, including provision for children identified as Gifted and Talented.

Extract: Garner, P and Davies, J D (2001) *Introducing SEN: A companion guide for student teachers*, **pp14–16. London: David Fulton.**

All teachers, and you will certainly be no exception to this, bring to the classroom a set of self-concepts, value systems, likes, dislikes, fears, expectations and so forth. Special education has always been something of an emotive topic, covering some difficult 'territory' and seeming to prompt strong feelings and controversy. Given that this is the case, we believe it is essential that you identify a personal standpoint or position. Put in fairly blunt terms, you need to establish what you stand for when it comes to SEN! A starting point for doing this is by exploring your own viewpoints – you will be able to make a more positive contribution to provision for SEN if you have interrogated yourself.

Consider the following reflective account, for instance. It is written by an experienced teacher, who now recalls her own schooldays:

> As a Girl Guide I remember visiting an institution where there were Down's Syndrome and autistic children. I had to spend two days with them for a badge and it was a real endurance test. I felt very uncomfortable because I had never been with such people. I think I looked down on them as lesser mortals, being thankful that I was not like them. They were outside my experience and I could not understand how the adults who cared for them could give them so much affection. Even as a Cadet Guider, when a girl with MS joined us I felt she was different and just could not treat her as a normal person. I think that some of my friends were also relieved when she left. I now have two good friends with MS and I know a dear boy with cerebral palsy. I think it is ignorance which breeds fear. (Garner *et al.* 1995, p. 12)

To what extent do you feel that the sentiments of the writer reveal something about her attitude to SENs? Is it fair to say that fear is bred from ignorance in respect of disabilities? Looking back on your own time as a pupil in school, do you recollect any similar experiences?

It is frequently the case that when certain people meet a disabled child or young person (especially if this is immediately obvious, for instance because of a visible disability) they can feel a sense of awkwardness in not knowing how to interact or respond. This might in part be due to the fact that a personal 'position' has not yet been developed by working through their own feelings about disability and 'difference'.

Some commentators have argued that one of the reasons at the heart of our response to 'difference' – which is often ambiguous or contradictory – is that we are sometimes confused by the 'meaning' of disability. An illustration of this can be found in Johnstone's observation that disabled people are 'either pathetic victims, arch villains or heroes. The stereotype of the disabled child is either that of the brave little lost boy/girl overcoming personal tragedy, or of the scheming malcontent determined to have revenge on society for the misfortune that has befallen him/her' (Johnstone, 1995, pp. 4–5). Put in terms of a child who has an SEN, teachers can feel both a sense of commitment to meeting his educational needs while, on other occasions, feeling somewhat threatened by the 'challenge' which the child presents.

When considering 'difference' – whether physical disability, or learning difficulty, it is often the case that we can slip easily into negative stereotyping. Hence, our view of what SEN means to us at this early stage in our development as a teacher can become polarised between views of children as 'able bodied' (positive) versus 'disabled' (negative), an illustration of which is provided below:

Able bodied	Disabled
Normal	Abnormal
Independent	Dependent
Good	Bad
Clean	Unclean
Fit	Unfit

While the polarities exemplified above are possibly extreme cases, there is no doubt that most teachers tend to develop a 'preferred' type of pupil – in respect of the way in which he approaches learning, his behaviour and so on. However, from this quite natural and understandable position it is only a very short step to negative labelling. Looked at from the standpoint of a classroom teacher, this kind of stereotyping can have serious consequences for the learner.

A further means of gaining an insight into this issue is by considering the range of names – mostly pejorative – which children in school use to characterise or describe others. Children who wear glasses, or who are overweight, children who appear to behave or learn in ways which are unusual, can all be subject to name-calling. A good example of this is the way that children whose behaviour in school is sometimes problematic may be described by a wide variety of unacceptable and stigmatising terms. These may range from 'nutters', 'mad' or 'mental' through to apparently more technical – though no less unsatisfactory – words such as 'disruptive' or 'pupils with problems'. It is entirely possible, too, that you may have heard such expressions being used by adults in other settings so deep seated is the fear of 'difference' in some people.

Analysis

Garner and Davies are explicit and outspoken about the fact that we, all of us, possess prejudices to those who display *difference*. They are clear that these prejudices are born out of ignorance and fear.

Personal response and reflection

What *type* of child do you prefer to teach?

Using the list of labels for stereotypes from Garner and Davies, above, mark where you are along the spectrum between each pair of labels, 5 being the midway point between the two labels. For example:

independent - - - - - - 7 - - - dependent

fit - - - 4 - - - - - - unfit

Reflect on your score and discuss with a colleague to compare views.

Why do you think you hold these views at this stage in your career?

One of the key implications of the work of Garner and Davies is that there is a need for extensive staff development opportunities for new and experienced teachers, to provide knowledge and understanding of what SEN categories exist and of how they can best make provision for them in their classrooms. Due to the changing nature of evidence, such training must be regularly reviewed to ensure current research findings are addressed in practice.

In order to work with SEN children effectively, it is helpful for teachers to be familiar with the broad SEN categories. These six areas (Hume, 2005) might be divided as follows, but with an understanding that some children will display needs in more than one category:

- sensory/motor difficulties;
- social/emotional difficulties;
- physical difficulties;
- behavioural difficulties;
- cognitive difficulties;
- speech and language difficulties.

While the term 'difficulty' is one used in the *Code of Practice* (DfES, 2001a), it perhaps serves to reinforce negative stereotypes. It would seem more appropriate in this age of personalised learning, to look at *all* children as having different needs, not difficult needs. How easy it is to internalise language and labels that then return to reinforce stereotyping attitudes in classroom practice.

What?

Before you read the following extract, read:

- Browne, A and Haylock, D (eds) (2004) *Professional issues for primary teachers*, Chapters 9–11. London: Paul Chapman Publishing.

These chapters provide you with an overview of the key debates surrounding SEN provision in the UK.

Extract: Hayes, D (2004) *Foundations of primary teaching*, 3rd edition, pp298–300. London: David Fulton.

Segregation, integration or inclusive education?

Segregation

Perhaps the major determinant of our success in educating children with SEN is our view about what should be done, and whereabouts it should come in the schooling process. The ideology behind segregation is that we are only responsible for children of 'normal' abilities and that specialist teachers should take the residue elsewhere, so we should resist changing our practice along inclusive lines. The term segregation not only applies to separate special schools, but also to segregation in mainstream schools, by special classes for the least able, groups permanently composed on ability lines, and withdrawal from class for 'extra help' on an ongoing basis. Recently, there has been a less visible form of segregation, when a classroom assistant is attached to one child and sits with him/her, accentuating the child's difference and progressively disempowering the child's opportunity to become an independent learner. There are, and have been shown to be, all sorts of practical problems with this sort of segregated education, which can be summarised thus:

- Because a group of children share some difficulties, it does not follow that they require the same kind of education provision.
- Children that are separated have limited access to a model of 'normal' classroom behaviour.
- When children are extracted from class they are falling further behind in the regular class work.
- The work they do under segregated conditions may not be related to the curriculum or the skills they need to access it; rather, it may be practice in basics unrelated to the curriculum or an excessive concentration on the use of worksheets.
- There is a lot of evidence to support the principle that children learn most effectively in group interaction, so the efficacy of 'one to one instruction' is questionable.

All children have varying abilities in different areas, so even if they benefit from individual instruction in one area it does not mean that they should be excluded from wider class and social activities. Even where children value separate treatment, there are stigmas attached to being seen as different by other members of the class. The practice of removal gives strong messages to the child about their perceived low standing, and damages their self-esteem and self-efficacy. Because of the above factors and the staffing costs involved, there has been a move towards more integrative and inclusive practices.

Activate your thinking!
Try to imagine what it must feel like to be treated differently from most other children.

Integration

Integration is the name given to the process whereby the formerly excluded were to be brought back into regular schooling, either moving from special to mainstream schooling, or by adopting class or group-based activities rather than individual 'remediation'. Through the 1980s 'integration' was the watchword, despite concerns as serious conceptual difficulties began to emerge. Pupils were to be integrated, or re-integrated, but the nature of the receiving school system remained immune to change. In other words, the basic assumptions behind the curriculum, assessment methods and teaching remained unaltered, the task was seen as fitting the child to the provision, not vice versa. As the school system had not been designed on the principles of inclusive assumptions, i.e. that it should be open to all members of the community, the practices it had developed over the period marked by segregation were not based on the widest needs in the community. The buildings were certainly inaccessible to anyone with problems with mobility, the curriculum was not necessarily relevant to all, and the practices of grading made it inevitable that a certain percentage of children would experience failure and the stigma that went with it. It was probably optimistic to believe that the ills of segregation could be alleviated by easing a few more disabled people into a system that was not designed with them in mind. From this point, educational policy started to move towards the principle of an inclusive system to meet all needs, though in some cases the practices that were used for integration have continued, and merely changed their name to inclusion!

Activate your thinking!
In what ways does integration benefit the mainstream population?

Inclusive education

Inclusive Education is best understood as an aim, aspiration or even a philosophy, rather than as a set of techniques that can be applied to a situation. It is a state that we move towards and a notion that regulates our efforts. Consequently, the school community is charged with offering education to all members of the community that it serves by modifying the way that all those involved work so that all needs are considered. Practices that tend to exclude would need to be eliminated in favour of more inclusive practices. Moving in an inclusive direction entails a problem-solving exercise on behalf of all those involved. For an account of a move towards a more inclusive ethos see the account of just such a problem-solving approach I applied to the development of an inclusive school (Thomas 1998). For the current statutory position about inclusion issues, see the DfES document, *Inclusive Schooling* (DfES 2001a).

Analysis

Hayes' extract raises a number of key areas for discussion, the most significant of which relates to segregation versus integration. This is particularly apt in the current climate of Workforce Reform (WAMG, 2003) and *Every Child Matters* (DfES, 2003c), in which a greater number of adults will be working alongside children in schools. The traditional deployment of teaching assistants has often been to work with children with identified learning needs – segregation in the classroom, according to Hayes. While, on the one hand, more adults working with children provide an opportunity for more needs-targeted teaching, it also holds the potential for further marginalisation within the mainstream setting as greater numbers of children work in isolation in small groups or one-to-one with an adult.

The integration of children with SEN into mainstream schooling is the practical response to policies to promote inclusion across all areas of education (DfES, 2001 b). Hayes' conclusions appear to suggest that this might have been poorly thought through, with the assumption that SEN children, who had been unable to attend their local primary school on the grounds that their difficulty precluded them from participating in the education, would now be welcomed back. Necessary adjustments would be made for them to participate. The criticism here seems to be, not with the principle of inclusion, but with the implied assumption that arrangements could be made to fit the children into the school environment. The *Index for Inclusion* (CSIE, 2000) project identified the need for the school community to change and develop from its fixed position to one which embraces and includes all learners. This project supports schools:

> in a process of inclusive school development by drawing on the views of governors, teachers and other staff, parents and carers, pupils and other community members. (Arthur *et al.*, 2005, p61)

The importance of an approach like this is that it provides for shared ownership and negotiation, where prejudices born from ignorance can be addressed through knowledge sharing, and where ultimately a shared environment can offer a safe learning culture to all who work in the school.

How?

Before you read the following extract, read:

- Hughes, P (2000) *Principles of primary education study guide*, 2nd edition, Chapter 9. London: David Fulton.

This chapter is a good illustration of how to translate policy into practice as a primary school teacher working to support SEN children.

Extract: DfES (2001a) *Code of practice on the identification and assessment of special educational needs*, **Fundamental Principles (1.5) and Success Factors (1.6). London: DfES.**

Fundamental principles
1:5 The detailed guidance in this Code is informed by these general principles and should be read with them clearly in mind:
- a child with special educational needs should have their needs met
- the special educational needs of children will normally be met in mainstream schools or settings
- the views of the child should be sought and taken into account

- parents have a vital role to play in supporting their child's education
- children with special educational needs should be offered full access to a broad, balanced and relevant education, including an appropriate curriculum for the foundation stage and the National Curriculum.

Critical success factors

1:6

- the culture, practice, management and deployment of resources in a school or setting[3] are designed to ensure **all children's needs are met**
- LEAs, schools and settings work together to ensure that any child's special educational needs are **identified early**
- LEAs, schools and settings exploit **best practice** when devising interventions
- those responsible for special educational provision take into account **the wishes of the child** concerned, in the light of their age and understanding
- special education professionals and **parents** work in **partnership**
- special education professionals take into account the **views of individual parents** in respect of **their child's particular needs**
- interventions for each child are **reviewed regularly** to assess their impact, the child's progress and the views of the child, their teachers and their parents
- there is close co-operation between all the agencies concerned and a **multi-disciplinary approach** to the resolution of issues
- LEAs make assessments in accordance with the **prescribed time limits**
- where an LEA determines a child's special educational needs, statements are **clear and detailed**, made within **prescribed time limits**, **specify monitoring arrangements**, and are **reviewed annually**.

Analysis

This document charts an important stage in the development of thinking about SEN provision (see Garner and Davies, 2001, p103 for a timeline of developments). As Hughes (2002) highlights, this Code of Practice elaborates upon the 1981 Education Act, which was groundbreaking in itself. It shifted away from labelling the child with terms such as *handicapped* or *subnormal* and placed the emphasis firmly upon the context in which the learner is working. This culture has required a considerable shift in perceptions and attitudes amongst teachers in mainstream schools. There is potential for conflict between established members of the profession who may be used to notions of segregation (either by educating children with SEN elsewhere, or separating them in the mainstream setting) and the newer recruits to teaching who have been immersed in an agenda focused around inclusion and integration. This may, perhaps, make for contradictory experiences for the student teacher on placement. While schools will be operating according to current requirements, individual teachers and staffroom conversation may reveal underpinning prejudices born out of an outdated understanding of SEN policy and practice. It will be important for you, as a new teacher, to evaluate comments made about children and privately reflect upon whether the comments are appropriate to a policy of inclusive practice.

The principles above resonate with the key themes explored in this book in that they enshrine, as good practice, partnerships with parents and listening to the views of the child. A concrete example of how this operates in practice is to be found in the Individual Education Plan (IEP). This document, if good practice is demonstrated, will involve:

- the child;
- support assistants working with the child;
- parents and carers;
- the class teacher;
- the special educational needs co-ordinator (SENCO).

If it is warranted, the IEP will develop as the basis for a statement of special educational need – this requiring the partnership to expand to include a wider range of experts such as healthcare workers and educational psychologists. This dialogue and sharing of expertise might be made easier and more informed if a school is operating as part of an extended school (*Every Child Matters*, DfES, 2003c) which facilitates multi-agency working and inter-professional dialogue.

Practical implications and activities

With reference to a school you have taught in, reflect (professionally) upon the following points with regard to SEN provision.

1. Look at the school's latest OFSTED report (**www.OFSTED.gov.uk**). Does the picture painted match your experience?
2. Review the SEN policy for the school. Can you identify a tendency to support segregation within school or inclusive integration?
3. Review an anonymous sample IEP from this school. With sensitive regard for the child's privacy, consider if you can identify the voices of the child and the parent or carer in the finished IEP.

Summary

In this chapter you have been challenged to confront your own views and prejudices, and to consider how these might influence your daily practice in the classroom. In so doing, it is anticipated that you will be able to reflect upon practice in schools, remembering that teachers will express private and informal views about the children they work with. SEN is an area subject to extensive and developing research and support. At this juncture, as we move to more fully integrated educational, health and social provision (*Every Child Matters*, DfES, 2003c), it is perhaps surprising to note that the TTA (2005) is proposing to pilot materials for student teachers in initial training that will require trainees to spend blocks of time in special schools as part of their studies. The views expressed in the opening paragraph of this chapter alluded to insecurity and a lack of confidence on the part of trainees when it comes to SEN, and policy developments and exemplars of good practice point to fully inclusive and integrated provision. Is it not contradictory to focus on the diminishing special school population, that might perhaps leave trainees with a set of coping strategies or 'tips' for teaching SEN children, when in fact it would be more valuable to support mentors in main-stream schools in structuring rich dialogue about inclusive practice in their schools. The dialogue might serve to move both parties forward, challenging prejudices along the way.

Further reading

Castle, F, Blamires, M and Tod, J (1998) *Implementing effective practice (IEPs)*. London: David Fulton.

Centre for Studies on Inclusive Education (CSIE) (2000) *Index for inclusion: developing learning and participation in schools*. Bristol: CSIE.

Soan, S (2005) *Achieving QTS. Reflective Reader: primary special educational needs*. Exeter: Learning Matters.

12 Acknowledging individual difference

By the end of this chapter you should have:

- further considered **why** it is important that teachers acknowledge and reflect on the boundaries of their professional relationships with children when providing pastoral support;
- reflected on **what** types of partnerships they establish with parents;
- analysed **how** you might develop your own strategies for working with parents and children to support pastoral and emotional development in schools.

Linking your learning

- Jacques, K and Hyland, R (2003) *Achieving QTS. Professional studies: primary phase*, Chapter 13. Exeter: Learning Matters.

Professional Standards for QTS
1.4, 1.6, 3.1.2, 3.2.4, 3.3.6, 3.3.9

Introduction

Adamson and Langley-Hamel in Jacques and Hyland provide a useful introduction into the parameters of the teacher's role and set this clearly within a whole-school context. This chapter concludes this section, and it is appropriate therefore that the focus is upon the needs of the whole child. While it has been appropriate to look at curriculum, assessment, classroom and behaviour management, for many primary teachers their role is complete when they have the opportunity to know the whole child. With this privilege comes considerable responsibility, as teachers find they need to employ a range of skills and emotional energy to support the pastoral needs of the children they are teaching. Many teachers enter the profession in response to a vocational calling and desire to work with young people yet, for some, the boundaries are hard to identify.

- Where does the role of teacher and parent overlap?
- How far should a teacher be friend and confidant(e)?

This chapter sets out to explore and discuss some of these dilemmas as we consider the pastoral role of the teacher. Teachers' legal and contractual obligations are discussed further in Section 4, although some requirements pertain to the teacher's pastoral role.

As you read this chapter, try to reflect on these two underpinning questions:

1. How does a teacher balance his/her own personal value systems when these are in conflict with a child's home environment?

2. Is the pastoral role of the class teacher more important than the educational role? (Blake, 2004, p112)

Why?

Before you read the following extract, read:

- **www.circle-time.co.uk**

This website provides an introduction to the principles underpinning circle time and some practical ideas on how to implement it.

Extract: Blake, G (2004) 'The primary teacher's responsibility for pastoral care', in Browne, A and Haylock, D (eds), *Professional issues for primary teachers*, pp104–106. London: Paul Chapman Publishing.

Health and safety

Pastoral care clearly involves ensuring – as far as is reasonable – the immediate physical safety of the pupils and the avoidance of any threats to their health. This aspect of the teacher's role complements that of 'health education' discussed in Chapter 14, where the emphasis is on promoting the children's long-term health and safety through their own learning. The teacher's concern for children's health and safety also operates within the legal framework of health and safety regulations (see Chapter 5).

Each school will have a fairly weighty tome entitled 'Health and Safety Policy' covering virtually every aspect of daily life in school. There will also be a designated health and safety officer on the staff to whom all concerns should be reported. Class teachers are required to exercise effective supervision of the pupils at all times and to know the emergency procedures in respect of fire, first aid and other emergencies. The 'effective supervision' question usually causes a great deal of discussion in staff rooms. Are the children allowed to stay in the classroom at playtimes without an adult in the room? And how do you manage a visit to the toilet when you have been on playground duty during break but must not now leave your class unattended for the five minutes you desperately need? Generally speaking there will be school procedures for such matters which it is advisable to follow, just in case a pair of scissors is waved around carelessly while you are absent from the classroom.

A primary school teacher who cares for the well-being of their pupils as a matter of course glances around the classroom each day wearing a metaphorical safety hat to check that the room is a safe place to be. This means, for example, checking that the escape doors are not blocked, that fire instructions are displayed clearly, and that there are no high objects liable to fall on heads or cables to trip over. Schools carry out regular fire drills and it is important to impose expectations for class behaviour at such times. These might be, for example, no talking, no running and lining up in a particular order. A culture where children follow oral instructions from their teacher without question obviously helps at such times. If the children trust the teacher to look after their well-being, any emergency procedures are likely to run smoothly.

Security and the screening of visitors is also taken very seriously in the present climate. There may be external classroom doors which have to be kept locked and a system of visitor passes which encourages children to challenge or report any adult not wearing the appropriate badge. This system is usually organized from the school office but staff and children need to be aware of the implications.

Other considerations under the safety umbrella include codes of practice for subjects with particular elements of danger such as science, physical education, design technology and information and communications technology. The subject co-ordinators are the sources of specialist advice on these matters. This is another area in which the enthusiasm of a trainee teacher or a newly qualified teacher to excite and engage the children may sometimes need to be curbed. Exciting pupil-activities which contain an unnecessary element of risk may have to be foregone in favour of something safe and boring!

Child protection
Possibly one of the weightiest responsibilities for a class teacher lies in the field – or minefield – of child protection. Whilst unfounded suspicions can lead to trauma for innocent families and the breakdown of the relationship between school and parents, it is important to remember that a failure to take action can, at its most extreme, lead to the death of a child. It is not uncommon for schools to be criticized for lack of knowledge and inefficient procedures when cases come to court. As with other sensitive areas a member of the school's senior management, often the headteacher, will be the designated teacher for child protection. This role involves undergoing training and understanding the local arrangements laid out by the Area Child Protection Committee (ACPC). In England, LEAs have drawn up their procedures following DfEE Circulars 10/95 and 11/95 (DfEE, 1995b; 1995c). These circulars provide government guidelines on protecting children from abuse. Many schools base their own policy on the United Nations Convention on the Rights of the Child and the principles of the 1989 Children Act (DoH, 1989).

The class teacher has a responsibility to protect children while they are in their care during the school day and on trips out of school. This includes reporting to the designated teacher any concerns, worries or suspicions that a pupil is suffering neglect, injury or abuse. Signs and symptoms to look out for include personality changes, physical problems such as tummy ache, tiredness, bruises and burns, and a general failure to thrive. During health education and other discussions teachers aim to provide children with the relevant information, skills and attitudes to resist abuse and to prepare for the responsibilities of adult life. It is important that if a child wishes to discuss sensitive matters at such a time, including a possible disclosure of abuse, the teacher does not promise confidentiality. This may compromise the responsibility to activate child protection procedures should anxieties arise. If a teacher becomes involved in preparing a court statement, this is done with the support of the school's designated teacher and a social worker within LEA guidance.

Physical contact
Government guidance for schools in England on the use of force to control or restrain pupils (DfEE, 1998b) sets the framework for school policies in this area. There are two main reasons for physical contact with children in school: first to offer comfort, reassurance and encouragement; and, second, to restrain them from some level of violence. It is very important that a teacher becomes acquainted with any school

guidelines on physical contact as they will offer protection to the teacher who may be put in a personally difficult situation by the consequences of well-meaning actions. In today's climate children who may have an axe to grind can make allegations that can leave the teacher in a very vulnerable position. Personal, social and health education lessons on topics such as 'personal space' and 'saying no to touching' will give children a positive context from which to make judgements.

School guidelines on physical contact usually give advice on:

- appropriate and inappropriate touches;
- gender issues;
- the avoidance of private situations;
- the fact that some children find any kind of physical contact disturbing; and
- physical restraint.

Physical restraint is only justified in the following circumstances:

- to defend yourself or others from assault;
- to stop an assault already happening;
- to stop a pupil inflicting serious harm on themselves; or
- to stop a pupil doing serious damage to property.

If possible, physical restraint should be left to senior management or designated members of staff who have had specific training on how to hold children in such cases. The best reaction is usually to remove the rest of the children from the scene of the violence if at all possible and to keep their normal routines going in a temporary venue. It is important to remember that vulnerable children may find incidents such as this particularly disturbing, so the teacher should plan a debriefing and a sharing of thoughts with the rest of the class. They could also talk through how they will react if such an incident happens again. Later in this chapter I will refer to some strategies for helping a child who may resort to violence if feeling under threat.

Analysis

Blake's chapter, while alerting teachers to the legislative framework in which pastoral support mechanisms need to operate, provides some important signposts to issues for primary teachers. In the heat and speed of the moment, a new teacher may not have the experience to know how to deal with a distressing pastoral matter. It is therefore essential that teachers are clear about school policies relating to pastoral issues, and know who to seek advice from within the school. On an emotional level, it is important that mechanisms are in place to support new teachers, with a clear line of advice and mentoring within the school. Obviously, experienced staff will have responsibility for seeking advice and support from other agencies if appropriate. Knowing how and when to seek external advice can be a cause of uncertainty for teachers. With the implementation of the extended schools agenda (*Every Child Matters*, DfES, 2003c) and closer interprofessional working, it could be hoped that this unease will be alleviated and more effective support for children provided.

Mosley's (1996) work illustrates one set of strategies for developing children's self-esteem and addressing pastoral needs. At the same time, she claims that the strategies promoted by circle time can lead to happier teachers who *will be less likely to leave their job* (2005). While there is no research evidence provided to support this claim, it appears to be the case that the methods she advocates are popular with primary teachers. There are critics of her work who, although supportive of her motives, warn of ethical issues that may arise around disclosure of information by the children (Pollard, 2005). However, her work is important and mirrors two themes from the Blake extract: the importance of establishing an environment in which children feel safe, and the support for communications skills and strategies that can be deployed to talk about affective or emotional issues.

The importance for learning of a safe and secure environment was discussed at length in section 1. It seems that it is similarly vital for children's pastoral and emotional well-being and development. Blake (2004, p112) refers to the importance of an anti-bullying policy and of children being trained to support and care for each other. It is often peers who can better understand and empathise with their classmate's issue, although, obviously, professional support and guidance may be needed if the issue warrants it.

Personal response and reflection

- How do you express your own personal need for emotional or pastoral support?
- What skills do you need to be able to seek this support?
- What are the key factors that allow you to be able to communicate this need?
- How does this relate to classrooms you have worked in?

What?

Before you read the following extract, read:

- Browne, A. (2004) 'Parents and teachers working together', in Browne, A and Haylock, D *Professional issues for primary teachers.* London: Paul Chapman Publishing.

This chapter provides an informative overview of the benefits and opportunities for working in partnership with parents.

Extract: Blandford, S (2004) *School discipline manual*, pp46–48. London: Pearson Education.

Effective teachers work in a consistent manner that will allow pupils to learn, and develop self esteem and self-confidence.

> *Good management allows the pupils to get a clear picture of what is going on and what is expected of them, and allows them to see more clearly the consistent consequences of their own behaviour, both desirable and undesirable.* (Fontana, 1994)

A few basic rules of good classroom management are suggested as follows:

- be punctual and well-prepared with appropriate material
- insist on full class co-operation, allocate teacher attention equally and be fair to all pupils and colleagues
- use the voice effectively – do not shout
- be alert to, and monitor and evaluate, what is happening in the classroom
- have clear and well-understood strategies for dealing with crises
- keep up-to-date with marking, and be consistent within the school marking policy
- make sure all promises are kept and deal with pupils' problems
- make good use of pupil- and teacher-led questions
- use a variety of teaching and learning styles
- wherever practical, delegate routine tasks to pupils
- organise the classroom effectively and ensure adequate opportunities for practical activities
- be conscious of your body language
- be consistent in the use of positive and negative reinforcers
- conclude the lesson successfully, summarise key points and dismiss the class in an orderly manner.

The majority of the above are also applicable to the management of corridors, play areas, dining rooms and halls.

The classroom
The term 'classroom' can be misleading when applied to schools. In the majority of schools, very few subjects are taught in a classroom with tables and chairs set out in regimented rows, with a white (or interactive) board at the front. An effective classroom seating plan is shown in Fig. 4.1, though this plan is determined by the size of the classroom. The teacher should consider the needs of each class. Varying the layout during the week will provide added structure and stimulation through the classroom setting. The majority of classrooms in primary and secondary schools have their own character as determined by the teacher. There are subjects in the school curriculum that are taught in spaces that are not rooms at all. 'Classroom' must be interpreted as the space in which pupils are taught.

Pupils need the right conditions to work. They must have access to books and equipment. Cramped classrooms are wholly inappropriate. Pupils also need to be able to see what the teacher is demonstrating. The design of the classroom also impacts on teachers. A teacher's personality will need to be considered when classrooms are assigned by management. The strain of working in an inappropriate space will affect the quality of teaching.

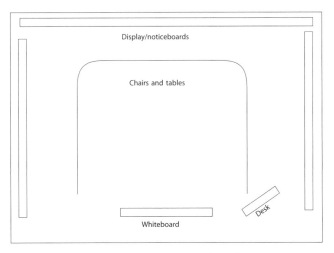

Figure 4.1 Classroom seating plan

In practice, the effect of the physical arrangements of the classroom will impact on discipline. As a resource, classrooms need to be utilised as effectively as possible. Primary school classrooms will need to accommodate sufficient equipment for all National Curriculum subjects, and provide ample space for 30 young pupils. The space must be appropriate to the subject and age group. Teaching music in a room designed for home economics does not inspire the teacher to teach and the pupils to learn. The space must reflect the teaching and learning styles of the teacher and subject. A drama teacher in a studio will have a different approach from that of a science teacher in a laboratory. For drama, the room will require black-out facilities to accommodate lights and storage for costumes and texts. A science laboratory will require benches, chairs, storage areas and a preparation room for the science technician to produce materials for each lesson.

Once in the classroom, pupils should have ready access to all materials and equipment, as required. Pupils should respect classrooms and equipment. They should also be taught to share. Pupils need to know and understand that they are members of a school community that respects its environment.

Having established the parameters within which both pupils and teachers work, there should be as few interruptions as possible to the period of teaching and learning. School notices and other messages should not be sent for delivery during lessons. Classrooms are busy places. Teachers need to be able to control timing effectively and smoothly; effective routines are essential for effective practice. It is important to provide pupils with a reference point to key words and classroom expectations.

Analysis

One of the key challenges for teachers supporting individual children will be when value systems held by the teacher and school may clash with those in the child's home. This will be acute if it involves pastoral matters. However, as Blandford stresses, positive relationships outside the family (in this case the school) have a beneficial effect on the child's ability to sustain relationships within the family. Thus, from a teacher's perspective, it is important to provide a safe but professionally distant space in which the child can form a positive relationship. This space must provide for a non-judgemental opportunity for the child to express pastoral or personal matters.

Blandford and Browne both allude to the importance of not distancing the parents and, where the child develops a close relationship with the teacher, there is always the danger that the parents may feel marginalised. Blandford stresses the fact that partnerships with parents can be challenging, and that the parents themselves may require support to be able to operate effectively and with confidence in a school setting where distressing matters may need to be discussed.

Practical activities and implications

Browne stresses the need for careful preparation prior to a parent consultation meeting.

1. Create a pen sketch of a child (fictitious or anonymous). This child has displayed bullying behaviour in school.

   - Make briefing notes for a meeting with the parents.
   - What are the key messages that you need to convey?
   - How are you going to ensure that the parent is able to contribute to the meeting?

2. With a partner, role play the consultation. What factors contributed to the success or failure of the meeting?

Summary

This chapter has explored some of the generic issues relating to supporting individual children, with a focus on pastoral support. It is clear that you, as a teacher, will require expert input and advice in this role but, importantly, you may need coping strategies to distance yourself from the issues.

Establishing a professional distancing framework will also allow you to retain some objectivity when analysing the issues. New teachers can find it emotionally demanding to separate out the personal and professional when handling pastoral situations. Pollard (2005) advocates the use of *bubble time* to provide a ring-fenced opportunity for the child to talk to the teacher. However, professional objectivity can be enhanced through focused observations of children. Creating a time when you, as teacher, can observe particular habits, behaviours and attitudes, over a period of time and in different contexts, can sometimes provide the space for reflection.

Further reading

Buck, M and Inman, S (1991) *Curriculum guidance no. 1: Whole school provision for personal and social development.* London: Centre for Cross-curricular Initiatives, Goldsmiths College.

Buck. M, Inman, S, and Tandy, M (eds) (2003) *Enhancing personal, social and health education: Challenging practice, changing worlds.* London: RoutledgeFalmer.

Pollard, A (2005) *Reflective teaching*, 2nd edition. London: Continuum.

Section 4: Becoming a professional

13 Professionalism, research and accountability

By the end of this chapter you should have:

- further considered **why** it is important that teachers engage in reflective, evidence-based research;
- reflected on **what** legislative requirements teachers need to work to;
- analysed **how** you might develop your own pedagogy in a way that is grounded in reflective practice.

Linking your learning

- Jacques, K and Hyland, R (2003) *Achieving QTS. Professional studies: primary phase*, Chapter 14 and 15. Exeter: Learning Matters.

Professional Standards for QTS
1.4, 1.5, 1.6, 1.7, 1.8, 3.3.1, 3.3.11, 3.1.3

Introduction

Education and the school workforce are facing radical change as a result of government consultation and legislation to improve the working conditions of teachers. This chapter sets out to explore teacher professionalism and accountability within this context. It draws upon material in Jacques and Hyland (2003, Chapters 14 and 15), and seeks to support discussion and reflection on key legislation and moral imperatives which influence the way teachers conduct their daily work.

Developments affecting the teaching profession over the past 20 years have involved moves to:

- make it an all-graduate workforce;
- assess teachers, in training and post-qualification, against a set of competencies and standards;
- standardise elements of curriculum content and delivery methods;
- introduce a greater variety of people to teaching by focusing on target groups (men and ethnic minorities);
- support flexible and employment-based options to train to teach;
- provide greater expertise and adult support in classrooms.

A range of views still exists about the role and status of teachers (Hayes, 2004). While there is an aura of sentimentalism about working with young children, and ideas of longer vacations and a short working day, the reality of the pressure to raise standards of academic performance, behaviour management and inspection regimes means that any sentimentality is short-lived. However, teaching is a public profession which will therefore reflect the values and needs of society.

Why?

Before you read the following extract, read:

- Pollard, A (2005) *Reflective teaching*, 2nd edition. London: Continuum.

Chapter 18 provides an interesting and challenging discussion about teaching and society.

Extract: Nixon, J (2002) 'Schoolteachers' legal liabilities and responsibilities', in Cole, M (ed) (2002) *Professional values and practice for teachers and student teachers*, 2nd ed, pp125–28. London: David Fulton.

Teachers' duty of care

There are three elements to the concept of a teachers' duty of care: the common law aspect, the statutory consideration; and the contractual obligation (for a discussion of this last element, see Chapter 8, where the 'Blue Book', the Schoolteachers' Pay and Conditions Document, was outlined in some detail).

The 'common law duty' was highlighted in *Lyes v Middlesex County Council* in 1962 (Local Government Review 1963) where the 'standard of care' expected of a teacher was held to be that of a person exhibiting the responsible mental qualities of a prudent parent in the circumstances of the school, rather than the home. It has been acknowledged that a teacher's duty of care to individual pupils is influenced by the subject or the activity being taught, the age of the children, the available resources and the size of the class. This can be clarified further by adding the proviso that, even though others may disagree, if it can be shown that the teacher acted in accordance with the views of a reputable body of opinion within the profession, the duty of care will have been discharged. The definition of the 'common law' duty of care may become even more sharply focused as progress is made to reduce the size of classes and with the establishment of the General Teaching Councils for England and Wales (GTCs).

Since September 2000 there has been established a GTC for England and a separate one for Wales; Scotland has had one since 1965. The GTCs have key powers over entry to the profession and the manner in which the profession conducts itself which will clearly impact upon individual teachers in relation to any issues that would fall into the category of misconduct. The GTCs will not have the powers that relate to pay and conditions; these issues will continue to be dealt with by the Review Body procedures outlined in the previous chapter.

With respect to the 'statutory duty of care', the Children Act 1989, Section 3, sub-section 5 defined the duty of care as doing 'what is reasonable in all circumstances of the case for the purpose of safeguarding and promoting the child's welfare'. Teachers who are entrusted with the care of children during the school day have this statutory duty. The

Children Act stresses the paramountcy of the wishes and needs of the child, reflecting the law's current more child-focused approach. Rather than the old-fashioned idea that a child was owned by its parents and this parental authority of property rights was delegated to teachers during the school day, the child's ascertainable needs and wishes should be taken into account by the teacher and considered in the light of the child's age and level of understanding. The teacher needs to assess the risk of harm that could arise to a child in particular circumstances, and to consider the safeguarding of the child and the promotion of the child's welfare and interest. This approach is clearly much more complex than the simplistic doctrine of the child as the property of the parents and demonstrates again how outmoded the term 'in loco parentis' has become.

It should also be noted that head teachers are required by the 'Blue Book' to carry out professional duties in accordance with the provisions of educational legislation, education orders and regulations, articles of government of the school, any applicable trust deed, any scheme of local management approved or imposed by the Secretary of State and any rules, regulations and policies laid down by the governing body under delegated powers or by the employing authority. In addition, a head teacher is also bound by the terms and conditions of any contract of employment, which means in totality that the head teacher is responsible for the internal organisation, management and control of the school.

If the concept of the 'duty of care' appears to be a complicated matter when it refers to activities within the school, it becomes ever more complex when a teacher is engaged in leading or assisting with activities off the school site, such as educational visits, school outings or field trips. The law on negligence is particularly significant here; the legal liability of a teacher or head teacher for any injury which is sustained by a pupil on a school journey or excursion would be dependent upon the three tests for negligence outlined earlier. If a child suffered an injury as a direct result of some negligence or failure to fulfil the duty of care, the employer of the teacher or head teacher would be legally liable. This is because employers have vicarious liability for the negligence of employees at work. Consequently where legal claims arise following an accident to a pupil, and there is a suggestion of negligence on the part of the teacher, the claim will most likely be made against the LEA as the employer of the teacher or the governing body in the case of Voluntary Aided, Foundation schools, sixth-form colleges or independent schools, if the teacher was, at the time of the accident to the pupil or student, working in the course of employment. It is, however, possible for teachers to be fined (see Chapter 8).

The standard of care required of a teacher is that which, from an objective point of view, can reasonably be expected from teachers generally applying skill and awareness of children's problems, needs and susceptibilities. Under health and safety legislation the law expects a teacher to do everything that a parent/carer with care or concern for the safety and welfare of his or her own child would do, bearing in mind that being responsible for up to 20 pupils or students at a time in an out-of-school activity is very different from looking after a family. The legal duty of care expected of an individual teacher can best be summed up by saying it is that which a caring teaching profession would expect of itself.

In practice this means that a teacher must ensure supervision of pupils throughout the journey or visit according to professional standards and common sense. Reasonable steps must be taken to avoid exposing pupils to dangers which are foreseeable and beyond those with which the particular pupils can reasonably be expected to cope. This does not imply constant 24-hour direct supervision while away on a residential field trip. The need for direct supervision has to be assessed by reference to the risks involved in the activity being undertaken. It is not enough merely to give instructions. The possibility that these instructions may be challenged by one or more of the pupils or students has to be taken into account, together with the risks the pupils may encounter if instructions are disobeyed. Equally pupils' *individual* levels of understanding and responsibilities have to be taken into account.

Where teachers believe that a journey or visit has not been adequately prepared or organised, they should not be expected to participate. It is important to note the terms in which the teacher's concern is expressed. If it is seen as a refusal to participate, in some circumstances this could be viewed as breach of contract or as an act of insubordination and could possibly lead to disciplinary procedures. The onus is on the teacher to demonstrate that there are proper professional and strategic reasons which give rise to the belief that there is a lack of preparation and organisation. Where the journey is one organised from within the school, responsibility for ensuring that proper preparation has been made and that proper supervision will be provided is ultimately that of the head teacher. Therefore it is the responsibility of head teachers to prohibit journeys and visits if they are not satisfied with the preparation and organisation of such journeys and visits.

Satisfying the duty of care absolves teachers from legal liability. However, sometimes accidents occur as a result of the fault of someone with no organising or supervising responsibility for the journey; for example, the bus company used for the trip. Should an accident occur where pupils and/or teachers sustain injury as a result of some defect in the vehicle, the bus company would of course be liable.

Some accidents are pure accidents, not reasonably foreseen and not the result of negligence on anyone's part; if no one is responsible then there can be no liabilities. Consequently liability goes with fault. In the case of a pure accident no one bears liability. Schools and LEAs will be covered in this eventuality by 'no-fault insurance'. Some LEAs act as loss adjusters for their own insurance procedures and settlement of a particular claim does not carry with it a notion of liability on the part of the LEA as employer. Recently an Appeal Court judge, deliberating on a case for damages following an accident, said something quite profound given the type of 'blame culture' we now encounter relentlessly in society. She said, 'Sometimes, somethings happen that are, quite simply, nobody's fault.' We would all do well to heed these words of wisdom before rushing to the law to attempt to apportion blame.

Analysis

Nixon's extract alerts teachers to the legislative frameworks that govern their daily working lives. These are also listed in Chapter 14 of Jacques and Hyland (2003). These frameworks are the mechanism by which society can ensure teachers are operating in a manner which supports its values. It is important to be vigilant, as policy and procedures with regard to teachers' working conditions change rapidly. Teachers are supported in this by the teaching unions and the General Teaching Councils (GTCs). The GTCs were introduced in 2000 and were charged with regulating the work of the teaching profession. They do this in two ways, through:

- the maintenance of high professional standards through regulation of the profession by members of the profession;
- the provision of evidence-led advice in order to maintain and develop expertise and systems within teaching. (Manning, 2004, p47)

Manning goes on to highlight some of the suspicions of and objections to the GTCs, which included an initial confusion about how the councils would work alongside or in opposition to the teaching unions. Given the immediate education history prior to the inception of the GTCs, many teachers were concerned that this may be another layer of bureaucracy and government regulation. To some extent the GTCs have been able to support a greater level of self-regulation and autonomy – this is evident in the award of full Qualified Teacher Status which comes from the GTCs and their involvement in conduct and competence matters. GTCs also have an overview of progression through the profession, from induction year, through threshold to Advanced Skills Teacher (AST) status. As new entrants to the profession, NQTs will have targets linked to the induction standards (TTA, 2003a). These will be monitored through the Career Entry and Development Profile (CEDP) (TTA, 2003b).

Practical activities and implications

Read the CEDP information for NQTs on the TTA website (**www.canteach.gov.uk**).

When you qualify you will need to identify areas of strength and areas for development. These will form the basis of an action plan during your induction year.

1. Based on your current experience, anticipate what you might like to focus on in your CEDP.

   - Identify three areas of strength that you might wish to develop further.
   - Identify three areas in which you feel less confident.
   - Ensure they link with the standards (TTA, 2003c).
   - Try to vary them so that they are not all linked to one area of the standards.

2. How might a school support you in achieving these during your first year of teaching?

What?

Before you read the following extract, read:

- Pollard, A (2005) *Reflective teaching*, 2nd edition, Chapter 16. London: Continuum.

Chapter 16 provides an interesting overview of the induction year.

Extract: Manning, R (2004) 'Teaching as a profession', in Browne, A and Haylock, D, *Professional issues for primary teachers*, pp44–46. London: Paul Chapman Publishing.

Can we recognize teaching as a profession?

Teaching is often described as a profession, but what does that mean for teachers and those who use their services? The reader is referred to Ozga and Lawn (1981), among others, for an in-depth discussion of the issue. Here we shall concern ourselves, in a simple form, with the most commonly agreed characteristics which identify a form of work as a profession:

1. It has a prestigious role that performs an essential service for its clients.
2. Admission is controlled by qualification requiring extensive training in skills and knowledge.
3. It has a high degree of autonomy.
4. It regulates the work of its own members to safeguard standards in the public interest.
5. It maintains and continues to develop an established body of special expertise and systems.

These characteristics can all be applied to a number of recognized professions: law, medicine, architecture and accountancy are all good examples. It is fairly easy to argue that the first two criteria have also applied to teaching for many years. Although teachers may disagree with the assertion that they are generally seen as a prestigious group within society (The *Guardian* website, GTCE/Guardian/MORI 2003 Teacher Survey), many parents still hold their own children's individual teachers in high esteem and public expectations of teachers have clearly increased over the years. It is on the last three points that, until recently, following the formation of the GTCs, the nature of teaching as a true profession has been disputed.

Autonomy?

In particular, teachers have complained that in their work they now have little autonomy, and that their professional judgement is undervalued. How much has the body of expertise been established, maintained and developed by those who work in teaching, and how much has been dictated by others outside the profession with other vested interests? Education in England and Wales has been highly politicized as evidenced by the significant number of additions and changes to legislation over the past 15 years. As has been argued in Chapter 1 of this book, since the introduction of the National Curriculum in 1988, much of the perceived body of special expertise – the skills and knowledge of the teacher – has been increasingly prescribed by central government, at times with apparently little regard to the voices of actual practitioners. The introduction of the National Literacy and Numeracy Strategies presumed to cover not just the content of the curriculum, but also the structure of the lessons and the teaching styles to be used.

Safeguarding standards?

In terms of regulation, teachers have become increasingly accountable to multiple external agencies. These include the DfES's prescribed curricula and initiatives, monitored by school inspection carried out by OFSTED. Other agencies of accountability are the LEA conducting its own monitoring and intervention, reports to parents and governors, the publication and comparison of national test results, and specialist intervention from social and health bodies, to name the major players. However, many of these agencies make little use of practising teachers in exercising judgements about teaching and learning.

Critical self-reflection has been emphasized in initial teacher training (ITT) in the past 20 years (Pollard, 1996). Many teachers' personal dedication to their work and the care of their pupils has made them constructively critical in evaluating their own performance and that of others. Teachers are awarded QTS following a process of initial teacher training. This usually involves some measure of professional judgement being made by qualified practitioners in schools where trainees serve their teaching practices. Yet, until recently, practising teachers have had no formal role in regulating standards of teaching after the award of QTS. Having attained QTS, teachers were registered with the DfES, but there was little formal recourse for dealing with conduct and competence issues beyond the school's governing body and the LEA/employer.

Maintaining and developing expertise?

In the area of maintaining and developing expertise, there have been no agreed expectations of continuing professional development. Opportunities for training and further development have varied from school to school and between LEAs. Until recently, classroom practitioners have had no formal role in developing and maintaining expertise and systems. However, LEAs are now making more use of, for example, advanced skills teachers (ASTs), leading mathematics teachers and others with specialist expertise to work alongside colleagues in other schools to improve the quality of teaching and learning.

Analysis

Manning notes that autonomy and self-regulation are two criteria listed as being essential if an occupation is to be deemed a *profession*. It is debatable whether the level of autonomy offered to teachers is sufficient to meet these criteria. However, it is also noted that the ability to develop expertise is another important element in professionalism. In this regard the profession may have much greater opportunities now than has been the case in recent times.

As an NQT you will be supported by an experienced, school-based colleague who will act as your mentor. If this relationship is resourced and professionally conducted, it can provide both partners with an opportunity to reflect on their own practice. As noted above, your development of expertise to effect change is a marker of professionalism. This small-scale and professionally intimate relationship can be the beginnings of evidence-based research which will impact on your practice in the classroom. Pollard (2005, p395) goes on to suggest that:

> reflection and mentoring help to inform and build a culture of professional learning. This is an important synergy, which leads to the construction of a learning community in the school.

There are also indications that teachers are being encouraged and supported to develop from this base, and to conduct classroom-based research to inform their practice. This can be seen in the resourcing of significant TTA projects, such as the teacher training resource bank (TTRB), the subject induction packs (SIPS) and the professional resource networks (IPRNs) for behaviour, citizenship and diversity. (Web references are given in the further reading section.) These projects bring together trainee teachers, teachers, teacher educators and researchers in editorially independent discussion forums with an opportunity to share practice and learn from experts. External research funding bodies are also becoming increasingly involved, providing resources for teachers to engage in classroom-based research.

In response to the 2003 OFSTED inspection framework, there is a much greater emphasis upon self-evaluation and review as a basis for assessing school performance. This is mirrored in the new teacher training inspection framework (OFSTED, 2005a), which also gives increased consideration to self-evaluation. LEAs are appointing senior staff to engage in this evaluation and review process. For example, an LEA in the south east is setting up research groups for teachers and LEA officers to work together in networked learning communities.

Personal response

Reflect on a classroom you have worked in.

Is there an issue, incident or question that left you pondering *why?* How might you translate this into an investigation which could be used to inform your practice?

How?

Before you read the following extract, read:

- George, R (2000) 'Starting your research project', in Herne, S, Jessel, J and Griffiths, J (eds) *Study to teach.* London: RoutledgeFalmer.

While the focus in this excerpt is on the submission of a piece of academic writing, the outlines and structures will be useful for all types of research in schools.

Extract: Clipson-Boyles, S (ed) (2000) *Putting research into practice*, pp2–5. London: David Fulton.

Research and practice: bridging the gap

It is also true to say that classrooms have been predominantly the sites for, rather than the beneficiaries of, research in the vast majority of cases. So why does this situation exist, when our common sense tells us that much of what is produced by educational researchers might make a difference to teaching and learning? There are three apparent reasons for the divide that are closely interlinked.

Lack of relevance

Firstly, research has not always seemed relevant to the classroom practitioner. There has tended to be a fragmented approach to research planning that has generated massive quantities of unrelated projects. The consequence of this is a lack of theory building through the accumulated knowledge of related or replicated studies, which would strengthen our existing knowledge. In some cases, studies on more obscure topics, although of interest and importance to the researchers, do not always appear to connect directly with classroom practice in ways that might make a difference to teaching and learning. That is not to say that small-scale, or minority interest studies should not exist. Indeed, they add to the rich multi-dimensionality of the educational research culture and, providing the limits on generalisability are understood, they can have much to offer. However, it is also true to say that there is a gap at the other end of the scale, with insufficient generalisable research to inform policy and practice.

Likewise, the links between research and development have been weak. All too often studies end, and the findings are left in a vacuum, the 'so what?' or 'what next?' factors failing to be addressed. This relates closely to the second reason for the research and practice divide.

Restrictive dissemination practices

Research has not always been disseminated in ways that are readable, accessible and usable to teachers. Full research reports are, of course, essential if studies are to be checked and replicated. Likewise, academic journals have an important part to play because the peer review process through which articles are scrutinised (before publication is approved or rejected) provides a systematic quality assurance process. However, the problem has been that many academics have fallen short of disseminating beyond this point. Some have argued that the Research Assessment Exercise (RAE; see Glossary) is to blame for this, the research being driven by the need to score points for funding rather than the needs of teachers and learners in the classroom. However, the fact remains that if a study is likely to be of interest and use to teachers, researchers have an ethical duty to ensure that it is disseminated for that audience, for example through professional publications, the development of resources and in-service training events. Indeed, it can be argued that planning for this should be included at the very start of the process when applying for funding, if we are to be truly accountable for the impact of our work (although clearly the actual outcomes will not be clear until the study is complete).

Divided communities

The third reason for the divide has been that research has been located as a separate activity or culture. In the past, teachers have rarely been consulted on what needs researching; they have been the subjects of studies rather than the instigators. It is unreasonable to expect all teachers to become researchers, although the reflective practitioner model is certainly something that all should adopt. However, it is perhaps time to consider other options that could strengthen the effectiveness of educational research. For instance, consultation partnerships when planning research, in-service dissemination of research, franchising of research among many individual schools linked by a coordinating researcher in the LEA or university, and so on. In other words, consultation and communication need to be considerably improved.

The changing culture of educational research

It is against this background that educational research is currently undergoing dramatic changes that offer exciting new opportunities and challenges for those working in education. These changes are probably due to four significant factors.

Teachers want research!

The recognition among a growing number of teachers that research can be relevant and useful to their everyday work means that there are greater expectations of researchers. Researchers now have to be more accountable for the quality of their work, and have a responsibility to report it appropriately.

The government wants research!

There has been a major shift by the present government towards developing evidence-based policy and practice at all levels. This is reflected by the commissioning and dissemination of research by the various education agencies, and the emphasis on teacher involvement. The government is also setting up systems to improve the sharing and communication of studies by extending the current research community into a more holistic and inclusive framework.

The research community is changing

For some time now, there has been a growing and vigorous debate taking place within the community of researchers about the quality, remoteness and cost-effectiveness of educational research (see Carnine 1995; Bassey 1996, 1997; Budge 1996; Hargreaves 1996). This has started to extend to other commentators such as Her Majesty's Chief Inspector of Schools, the Teacher Training Agency (TTA) and the Department for Education and Employment (DfEE). News items have also meant that the debate is also starting to reach the ears of teachers! Two reviews took place in 1998 to investigate the state of educational research in Britain. One was commissioned by the Office for Standards in Education (OFSTED) (Tooley and Darby 1998) and the other by the DfEE; the latter was undertaken by the Institute for Employment Studies (Hillage *et al.* 1998). Although very different in character and methodology, both studies found that educational research was currently having little impact on, or relevance to, policy and practice (although it was agreed that this is an extremely difficult thing to isolate and measure). These two reports make interesting reading and should be studied closely by all who are interested in the current debate.

Changing research practices

There is an ever increasing diversity of approaches to research methods and methodologies. Some, particularly those who are committed to a very specific paradigm, see this as problematic. Others see this as tremendously beneficial because it means that education is being examined in different ways from a rich variety of perspectives, which gives a multifaceted picture of what is happening in schools. In the early days of educational research, traditional scientific methods (quantitative) were usually used to measure specific variables that could be isolated (e.g. intelligence, reading age, etc.). However, some would argue that the social nature of education renders it almost impossible to isolate variables in the way that scientists might do in a laboratory. This resulted in the growth of more ethnographic approaches, which created what is still sometimes called the quantitative/qualitative divide. In reality, each of these categories can be further subdivided into a fascinating number of different approaches. Many researchers (although by no means all) are starting to recognise that rather than competing, the two paradigms can be mutually beneficial. Scientific checks can ensure that we are not making unrepresentative claims, and ethnographic insights can add more depth to otherwise two-dimensional number-crunching. The debate about approach is important, but it is underpinned by the equally significant argument about quality. Unbiased sampling, triangulation, clear descriptions of method and methodology and transparent selection of data for reporting are all required if objectivity and integrity are to be assured. And even in more personal studies where subjectivity is part of what is being explored, that should be clear to the reader. (Details of terminology are provided in the Glossary if required.)

This new culture offers tremendous scope for positive change and development as the ownership of research shifts towards a more inclusive framework. An important theme running through this book is the implications of this for teaching and learning.

Analysis

Clipson-Boyles' edited collection is designed to support teachers to see the links and applications of research to classroom practice. The whole book provides a range of case study exemplars across a spectrum of generic issues and curriculum-specific areas. The three introductory remarks she makes are significant in the context of impending and new developments in education. For teachers, research has been seen as irrelevant, inaccessible and unrelated to classroom practice. However, as research now begins to gain favour among classroom practitioners, it is important to consider possible issues that this raises. The increasing shift to work-based and flexible or distance-learning training routes means that fewer new teachers will have access to the pool of research expertise that exists in the higher education (HE) sector. The consequences, if planned in a systematic and strategic way, will have positive benefits for school and HE staff. Tabberer (2004) called for members of this community to help *redesign the Titanic before she sails*. It will no longer be feasible for HE staff to remain static within their institutions and, increasingly, it will be the case that their expertise could be utilised in schools to support reflective, evidence-based practice alongside initial teacher training and professional development work. In order to enhance quality and sustainability, this context-based development will need to be underpinned by reflective practice. I would argue that HE-based staff are very well placed to support the development of reflective practice. According to McIntyre (1993) there are three levels of reflection: technical, practical, and emancipatory or critical. It is in the last of these that school staff may well require the support of an experienced research facilitator who can support the development of a reflective learning community. This in turn could be linked to accreditation leading to a Master's degree or further qualifications.

Summary

This chapter has been about challenging you to see your role as class teacher within a series of contexts and networks. Teachers work in an environment which is full of people, but it can be a lonely and isolating experience.

Within your school you will have a class, a year group, a key stage, a playground, a school gate and a staffroom. Each of these provides a context in which there are rules for belonging and where identities are shaped. As a teacher you will be part of a school, a cluster and an LEA. You will also be part of a wider set of communities that influence and govern your work in school. Reflective practice is about using questions to explore how these communities operate and interact, and making changes to your teaching as a result. But, as a member of these interlocking communities, you too are influencing change in the world of education. Your thoughts and questions will prompt a response and generate activity that, ultimately, will make a difference.

Further reading

Cole, M (2005) (ed) *Professional values and practice. Meeting the standards*, 3rd edition. London: David Fulton.
GTCE (2001) *Professional learning framework*. London: GTCE.
GTCE (2002) *Professional code for teachers*. London: GTCE.
Kyriacou, C (1991) *Essential teaching skills*. Cheltenham: StanleyThornes.
www.multiverse.org
www.behaviour4learning.ac.uk
www.citized.ac.uk
www.ttrb.ac.uk

And a final thought …

> *Only a teacher?*
> *Thank God I have a calling to the greatest profession of all! I must be vigilant every day lest I lose one fragile opportunity to improve tomorrow.*
> Ivan Welton Fitzwater

References

Arthur, J, Davison, J and Lewis, M (2005) *Professional Values and Practice.* London: RoutledgeFalmer.

Assessment Reform Group (1999) *Beyond the Black Box.* Cambridge: Cambridge University School of Education.

Barnes, D (2002) 'Knowledge, communication and learning', in Pollard, A (ed) *Readings for Reflective Teaching.* London: Continuum.

Bastide, D (1999) *Co-ordinating RE across the Primary School.* East Sussex: Falmer Press.

Bearne, E (ed) (1996) *Differentiation and Diversity.* London: Routledge.

Bennett, N, Desforges, C, Cockburn, A and Wilkinson, B (1984) *The Quality of Pupil Learning Experiences.* London: Lawrence Erlbaum Associates.

Bigger, S and Brown, E (eds) (1999) *Spiritual, Moral, Social and Cultural Development.* London: David Fulton.

Black, P, Harrison, C, Lee, C, Marshall, B and Wiliam, D (2002) *Working Inside the Black Box: Assessment for Learning in the Classroom.* London: Nfer Nelson.

Blair, M (2002) 'Education for All', in Cole, M (ed) *Professional Values and Practice for Teachers and Student Teachers*, 2nd edition. London: David Fulton.

Blake, G (2004) 'The primary teacher's responsibility for pastoral care', in Browne, A and Haylock, D (ed) *Professional Issues for Primary Teachers.* London: Paul Chapman Publishing.

Blandford, S (2000) 'Managing positive behaviour', in Clipson-Boyles, S (ed) *Putting Research into Practice in Teaching and Learning.* London: David Fulton.

Blandford, S (2004) *School Discipline Manual.* London: Pearson Education.

Brown, A and Furlong, J (1996) *Spiritual Development in Schools: Invisible to the Eye.* London: The National Society.

Brown, A and Seaman, A (2001) *Feeding Minds and Touching Hearts: Spiritual Development in the Primary School.* London: National Society.

Browne, A (2004) 'Parents and teachers working together', in Browne, A and Haylock, D (eds) *Professional Issues for Primary Teachers.* London: Paul Chapman Publishing.

Bruner, J S (1986) *Actual Minds, Possible Worlds.* Cambridge, MA: Harvard University Press.

Buck, M and Inman, S (1991) *Curriculum Guidance No. 1: Whole School Provision for Personal and Social Development.* London: Centre for Cross-curricular Initiatives, Goldsmiths College.

Buck, M, Inman, S and Tandy, M (eds) (2003) *Enhancing Personal, Social and Health Education: Challenging Practice, Changing Worlds.* London: Routledge Falmer.

Burns, S and Lamont, G (1995) *Values and Visions.* London: Hodder and Stoughton.

Castle, F, Blamires, M and Tod, J (1998) *Implementing Effective Practice (IEPs).* London: David Fulton.

Centre for Studies on Inclusive Education (CSIE) (2000) *Index for Inclusion: Developing Learning and Participation in Schools.* Bristol: CSIE.

Clarke, S (2001) *Unlocking Formative Assessment: Practical Strategies for Enhancing Pupils' Learning in the Primary Classroom*. London: Hodder and Stoughton.

Claxton, G (1999) *Wise Up: the Challenge of Lifelong Learning*. London: Bloomsbury.

Claxton, G (2002) 'Learning and the development of resilience', in Pollard, A (ed) *Readings for Reflective Teaching*. London: Continuum.

Claxton, G (1997) **www.knowdrama.com/articles/cynicism** (accessed 30 June 2005).

Clipson-Boyles, S (ed) (2000) *Putting Research into Practice*. London: David Fulton.

Coles, R (1986) *The Moral Life of Children*. New York: First Atlantic Press.

Cole, M (ed) (2002) *Professional Values and Practices for Teachers and Student Teachers*, 2nd edition. London: David Fulton.

Dadds, M (2002) 'The "hurry-along" curriculum', in Pollard A (ed) *Readings for Reflective Teaching*. London: Continuum.

DES (1988) *Education Reform Act*. London: HMSO.

DES (1989) *National Curriculum: From Policy to Practice*. London: DES.

DES (1989) *Discipline in Schools, Report of the Committee of Enquiry, chaired by Lord Elton*. London: HMSO.

Desforges, C (ed) (1995) *An Introduction to Teaching: Psychological Perspectives*. London: Blackwell.

DfE (1993) *The Initial Training Of Primary School Teachers: New Criteria for Courses*. Circular 14/93. London: DfE.

DfEE/QCA (1999) *The National Curriculum: Handbook for Primary Teachers in England Key Stages 1 and 2*. London: DfEE/QCA.

DfES (1996b) *The Secretary of State's Guidance on Pupil Behaviour and Attendance*. London: DfES.

DfES (1998) *Requirements for Courses of Initial Teacher Training: High Status, High Standards*, Circular 4/98. London: DfES.

DfES (1998) *The Literacy Strategy*. London: DfES.

DfES (1999a) *The Numeracy Strategy,* London: DfES.

DfES (2001a) *Code of Practice on the Identification and Assessment of Special Educational Needs*. London: DfES.

DfES (2001b) *Inclusive Schooling*. London: DfES.

DfES (2002) *Education Act*. London: DfES.

DfES (2003a) *Five Year Strategy for Children and Learners*. London: DfES.

DfES (2003b) *The Primary Strategy*. London: DfES.

DfES (2003c) *Every Child Matters*. London: DfES.

DfES (2003d) *Using the National Healthy School Standard to Raise Boys' Achievement*. London: DfES.

DfES (2004a) *Learning and Teaching in the Primary Years. Professional Development Resources*. London: DfES.

DfES (2004b) *The Children Act*. London: DfES.

DfES (2004c) *Behaviour in the Classroom: A Course for Newly Qualified Teachers*. **www. standards.dfes.gov.uk**

Doddington, C (1996) 'Grounds for differentiation. Some values and principles in primary education considered', in Bearne, E (ed) *Differentiation and Diversity*. London: Routledge.

Edwards, D and Mercer, N (2002) 'Classroom discourse and learning', in Pollard A (ed) *Readings for Reflective Teaching.* London: Continuum.

English, E and Newton, L (2005) *Professional Studies in the Primary School.* London: David Fulton.

English, E (2005) 'Teachers as professionals: The background', in England, E and Newton, L *Professional Studies in the Primary School.* London: David Fulton.

Erricker, C and Erricker, J (2000) *Reconstructing Religious, Spiritual and Moral Education.* London: RoutledgeFalmer.

Filer, A and Pollard, A (2002) 'The myth of objective assessment', in Pollard, A (ed) *Readings for Reflective Teaching.* London: Continuum.

Gaine, C (1995) *Still No Problem Here.* Stoke on Trent: Trentham Books.

Gardner, H (1997) **www.knowdrama.com/articles/cynicism** (accessed 30 June 2005).

Gardner, H (1985) *Frames of Mind: Theory of Multiple Intelligences.* London: Paladin Books.

Garner, P and Davies, J D (2001) *Introducing Special Educational Needs.* London: David Fulton.

George, R (2000) 'Starting your research project', in Herne, S, Jessel, J and Griffiths, J (eds) *Study to Teach.* London: Routledge.

Goleman, D (1996) *Emotional Intelligence Why it Matters More than IQ.* London: Bloomsbury.

Grainger, T and Kendall-Seatter S (2003) 'Drama and spirituality: Reflective connections'. *International Journal of Children's Spirituality,* 8, 1.

Griffiths, J (2000) 'Presenting your work orally', in Herne, S, Jessel, J and Griffiths, J (ed) *Study to Teach.* London: Routledge.

Grossman, H (2004) *Classroom Behaviour Management for Diverse and Inclusive Schools,* 3rd edition. Oxford : Rowman and Littlefield.

GTCE (2001) *Professional Learning Framework.* London: GTCE.

GTCE (2002) *Professional Code for Teachers.* London: GTCE.

Hay McBer (2000) *Research into Teacher Effectiveness: A Model of Teacher Effectiveness.* London: DfEE.

Hay, D and Nye, R (1998) *The Spirit of the Child.* London: HarperCollins.

Hayes, D (1997) 'Teaching competencies for Qualified Primary Teacher Status in England', in *Teacher Development,* 1, 2.

Hayes, D (2004) *Foundations of Primary Teaching,* 3rd edition. London: David Fulton.

Headington, R (2003) *Monitoring, Assessment, Recording, Reporting and Accountability: Meeting the Standards,* 2nd edition. London: David Fulton.

HMI (1994) 'Characteristics of Good Practice', in Pollard, A and Bourne, J (eds) *Teaching and Learning in the Primary School.* Oxford: OUP.

Houghton, S, Whedell, K, Jukes, R and Sharpe, A (1990) 'The effects of limited private reprimands and increased private praise on classroom behaviour in four British secondary school classes'. *British Journal of Educational Psychology,* 60, 3.

Hughes, P (2002) *Principles of Primary Education Study Guide,* 2nd edition. London: David Fulton.

Hume, T (2005) 'Different needs and different responses', in English, E and Newton, L (eds) *Professional Studies in the Primary School.* London: David Fulton.

Inman, S, Buck, M and Burke, H (1998) *Assessing Personal and Social Development: Measuring the Unmeasurable.* London: RoutledgeFalmer.

Jessel, J (2000) 'Study: some guiding principles', in Herne, S, Jessel, J and Griffiths, J (ed) *Study to Teach.* London: Routledge.

Kendall, S (2000) 'Establishing and maintaining professional working relationships', in Herne, S, Jessel, J and Griffiths, J (eds) *Study to Teach.* London: Routledge.

Kounin, J S (1970) *Discipline and Group Management in Classrooms.* New York: Holt Rhinehart & Winston.

Kyriacou, C (1991) *Essential Teaching Skills.* Cheltenham: Stanley Thornes.

Laslett, R and Smith, C (2002) 'Four rules of class management', in Pollard, A (ed) *Readings for Reflective Teaching.* London: Continuum.

Leont'ev, A N (1981) *Problems of the Development of Mind.* Moscow: Progress Publishers.

Lewisham Education Service (1999) *SMSC Providing for Spiritual, Moral, Social and Cultural Development of Pupils.* London: Continuum.

Macready C (2005) 'Using data to narrow the achievement gap.' **www.standards.dfes.gov.uk**

Maden, M (2002) 'Social circumstances in children's experience of exclusion', in Pollard, A (ed) *Readings for Reflective Teaching.* London: Continuum.

Manning, R (2004) 'Teaching as a Profession', in Browne, A and Haylock, D (eds) *Professional Issues for Primary Teachers.* London: Paul Chapman Publishing.

Mathieson, K and Price, M (2001) *Better Behaviour in Classrooms: A Course of INSET Materials.* London: RoutledgeFalmer.

McIntyre, D (ed) (1993) *Mentoring.* London: Kogan Page.

McNamara, S and Moreton, G (1997) *Understanding Differentiation.* London: David Fulton.

Mercer, N (2002) 'Culture, context and the appropriation of knowledge', in Pollard, A (ed) *Readings for Reflective Teaching.* London: Continuum.

Merrett, F and Tang, W M (1994) 'The attitudes of British primary schools to praise, rewards, punishments and reprimands'. *British Journal of Educational Psychology,* 64, 1.

Mortimore, P, Sammons, P, Stoll, L, Lewis, D, and Russell, E (1994) 'Teacher expectations', in Pollard, A and Bourne, J (eds) *Teaching and Learning in the Primary School.* London: Routledge.

Mosley, J (1996) *Quality Circle Time,* Cambridge: LDA.

Mosley, J **www.circle-time.co.uk** (accessed July 2005).

Newton, L (2005) 'The individual in the primary classroom', in English, E and Newton, L (eds) *Professional Studies in the Primary School.* London: David Fulton.

Nixon, J (2002) 'Schoolteachers' legal liabilities and responsibilities', in Cole, M (ed) *Professional Values & Practice for Teachers and Student Teachers,* 2nd edition. London: David Fulton.

Northern Ireland Department of Education (1999) *The Teacher Education Partnership Handbook.* Belfast: Northern Ireland Department of Education.

OFSTED (2003a) *Handbook for Inspecting Primary and Nursery Schools.* London: OFSTED.

OFSTED (2003b) *Inspecting Schools: Framework for Inspecting Schools.* London: OFSTED.

OFSTED (2004) *Promoting and Evaluating Pupils' Spiritual, Moral, Social and Cultural Development.* London: OFSTED.

OFSTED (2005a) *Framework for the Inspection of Initial Teacher Training for inspections from September 2005.* London: OFSTED.

OFSTED (2005b) *Managing Challenging Behaviour.* London: OFSTED.

Oldham, J (2005) 'Consideration for Pupils as Learners', in Cole, M (ed) *Professional Values and Practice: Meeting the Standards*, 3rd edition. London: David Fulton.

Pollard, A and Bourne J (eds) (1994) *Teaching and Learning in the Primary School.* London: RoutledgeFalmer.

Pollard, A (1997) *Reflective Teaching in the Primary School*, 3rd edition. London: Cassell.

Pollard, A (ed) (2002) *Reading for Reflective Teaching.* London: Continuum.

Pollard, A (2005) *Reflective Teaching*, 2nd edition. London: Continuum.

Pollard, A and Tann, S (1993) *Reflective Teaching in the Primary School*, 2nd edition. London: Cassell.

Powell, S and Tod, J (2004) *Research Evidence in Education.* London: EPPI Centre, Social Science Research Unit, Institute of Education.

QCA (1998a) *Education for Citizenship and the teaching of Democracy in Schools*, Crick Report. London: QCA.

QCA (1998b) *The National Curriculum: Handbook for Primary Teachers in England.* London: HMSO.

Rogers, C R (1969) *Freedom to Learn.* New York: Merrill.

SCAA (1997) *Findings of the Consultation on Values in Education and the Community.* London: HMSO.

Smith, J (2004) 'Gender issues in primary schools', in Browne, A and Haylock, D (ed) *Professional Issues for Primary Teachers.* London: Paul Chapman Publishing.

Soan, S (2005) *Achieving QTS: Reflective Reader Primary Special Educational Needs.* Exeter: Learning Matters.

Socialist Review (1994)

Stierer, B, Devereux, J, Gifford, S, Laycock, E and Yerbury, J (1993) *Profiling, Recording, and Observing: A Resource Pack for Early Years.* London: Routledge.

Tabberer, R (2004) *Speech to UCET conference, November 2004.*

Tann, S (1995) 'Organizing the learning experience', in Desforges, C (ed) *An Introduction to Teaching: Psychological Perspectives.* Oxford: Blackwell Publishers.

Thatcher (1999) *Spirituality and the Curriculum.* London: Continuum.

Tickle, L (1996) 'Reflective teaching: Embrace or illusion?', in McBride, R (ed) *Teacher Education Policy: Some Issues Arising from Research and Practice.* London: Falmer Press.

TTA (2003a) *The Induction Standards.* London: TTA.

TTA (2003b) *The Career Entry and Development Profile.* London: TTA.

TTA (2003c) *Qualifying to Teach: The Professional Standards for Qualified Teacher Status and Requirements for Initial Teacher Training.* London: HMSO.

TTA (2005) *Qualifying to Teach: Handbook for Guidance.* London: HMSO.

TTA (2005) *NQT Survey.* **www.tta.gov.uk**

Vygotsky, L S (1978) *Mind in Society: The Development of Higher Psychological Processes.* Cambridge, MA: Harvard University Press.

WAMG (2003) 'Guidance for schools on carer supervision'. **www.teachernet.gov.uk**

Wenham, M (1995) 'Developing thinking and skills in the arts', in Moyles, J (ed) *Beginning Teaching: Beginning Learning.* Maidenhead: OUP.

Woods, P (1996) 'Teachers and classroom relationships', in Pollard, A (ed) *Readings for Reflective Teaching.* London: Continuum.

Worton, C (2005) 'Classroom approaches and organisation', in English, E and Newton, N (eds) *Professional Studies in the Primary School.* London: David Fulton.

Wragg, E C and Wood, E K (1984) 'Teachers' first encounters with their classes', in Wragg, E C (ed) *Classroom Teaching Skills.* London: Croom Helm.

Wright (2000) *Spirituality and Education.* London: RoutledgeFalmer.

www.behaviour4learning.ac.uk

www.citized.ac.uk

www.multiverse.org

www.routledgefalmer.com/pdf/Behaviour.pdf

www.teachernet.gov.uk

www.ttrb.ac.uk

Index